Diabetes Management

and

Treatment

Learn How to Better Control Diabetes

and

Minimize Its Effects

Ron Kness

Published by:

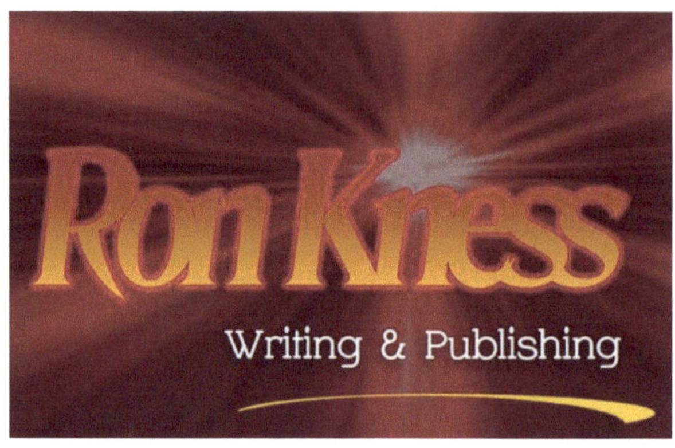

https://ronknesswriting.com

Ron Kness

Queen Creek, AZ

United States of America

For

Healthy Lifestyle Newsletter – Diabetes Management

https://healthylifestylenewsletter.com/diabetes

ISBN: 9798728396536

Disclaimer

This publication is for informational purposes only and is not intended as medical advice. Medical advice should always be obtained from a qualified medical professional for any health conditions or symptoms associated with them.

Every possible effort has been made in preparing and researching this material. We make no warranties with respect to the accuracy, applicability of its contents or any omissions.

See your healthcare professional before starting any diet, health or exercise program!

Contents

Type One Diabetes Versus Type Two Diabetes Explained

If someone is asked to describe their health, they'll usually say that they're diabetic. Most people don't mention whether they have Type one or two diabetes. Both conditions cause the body to struggle with glucose storage and usage.

Glucose is used by the body to create energy, and diabetics have impaired ability to collect the free glucose in the bloodstream, starving the body's cells of needed energy. The two main types of diabetes have many similarities, but they are different diseases.

Let's differentiate between them.

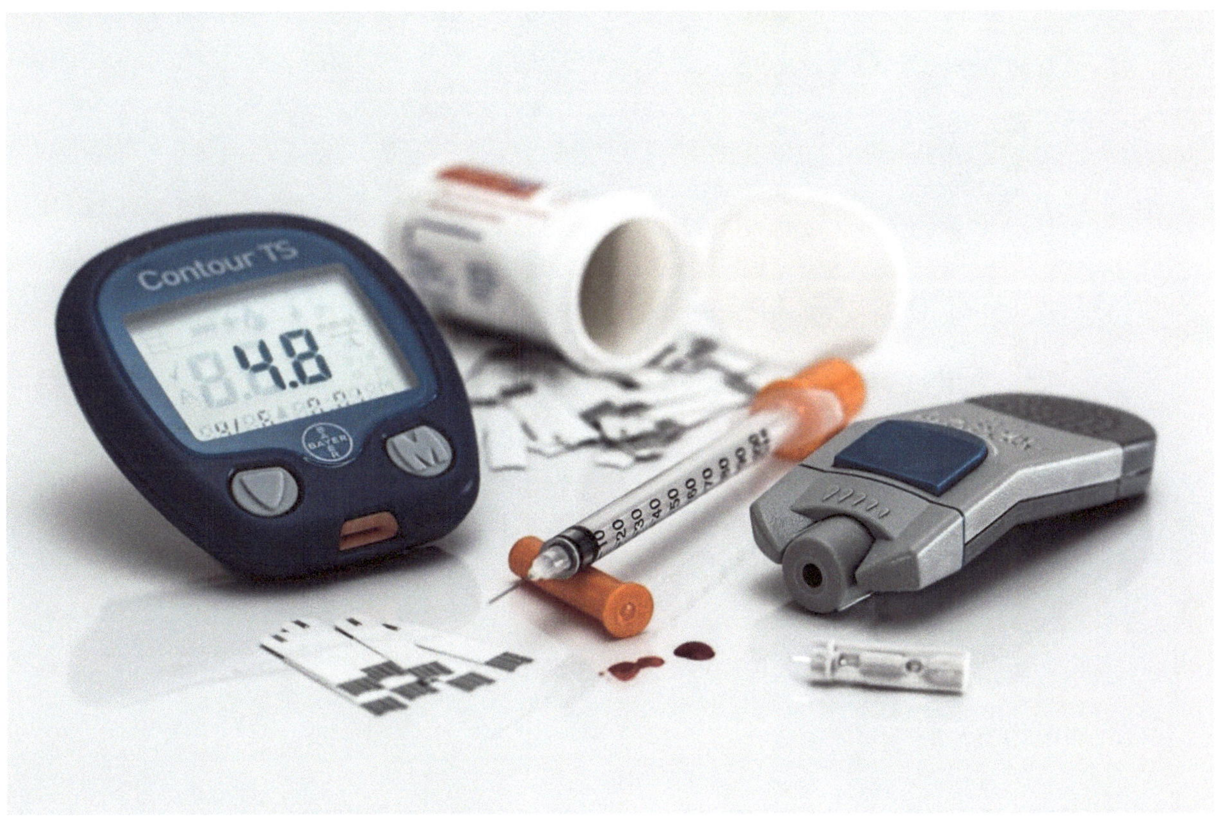

Diabetes Type Two (T2D)

T2D is the most common, affecting 90 to 95% of Americans with diabetes. It occurs most often in mature individuals over the age of 45, but teenagers, young adults, and children are being affected, too.

Diabetes Type Two is when your body can still produce insulin, but the insulin produced is much less useful. You actually become resistant to this hormone that the body needs to regulate your blood glucose levels.

Risk Factors

Ethnicity plays a huge role in the risk of developing T2D. According to Harvard Medical School, Asian Americans, African Americans, Native Americans, and Hispanics are more likely to develop T2D.

Genetics is another risk factor. Inheriting certain genes makes you three times more likely to develop diabetes. The main culprit is lipids inside the pancreatic B cell membranes, which cause blockage of the process of storing and converting glucose to energy.

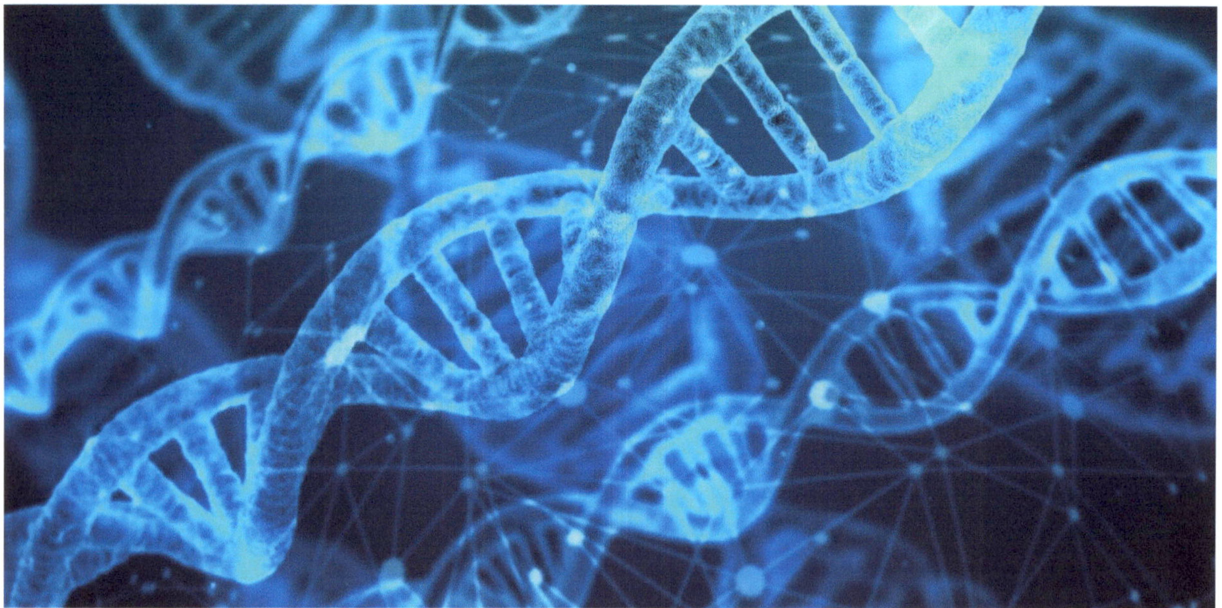

Obesity is another risk factor for anyone with a body mass index (BMI) of 25 or higher as well as smoking which increases your risk of developing T2D by 30 to 40%.

Other factors include:

- A lack of exercise and an unhealthy diet also increases your risk.
- Environmental factors certainly contribute risk.
- T2D might even be the consequence of having too little vitamin D.

And finally, age certainly plays a big role.

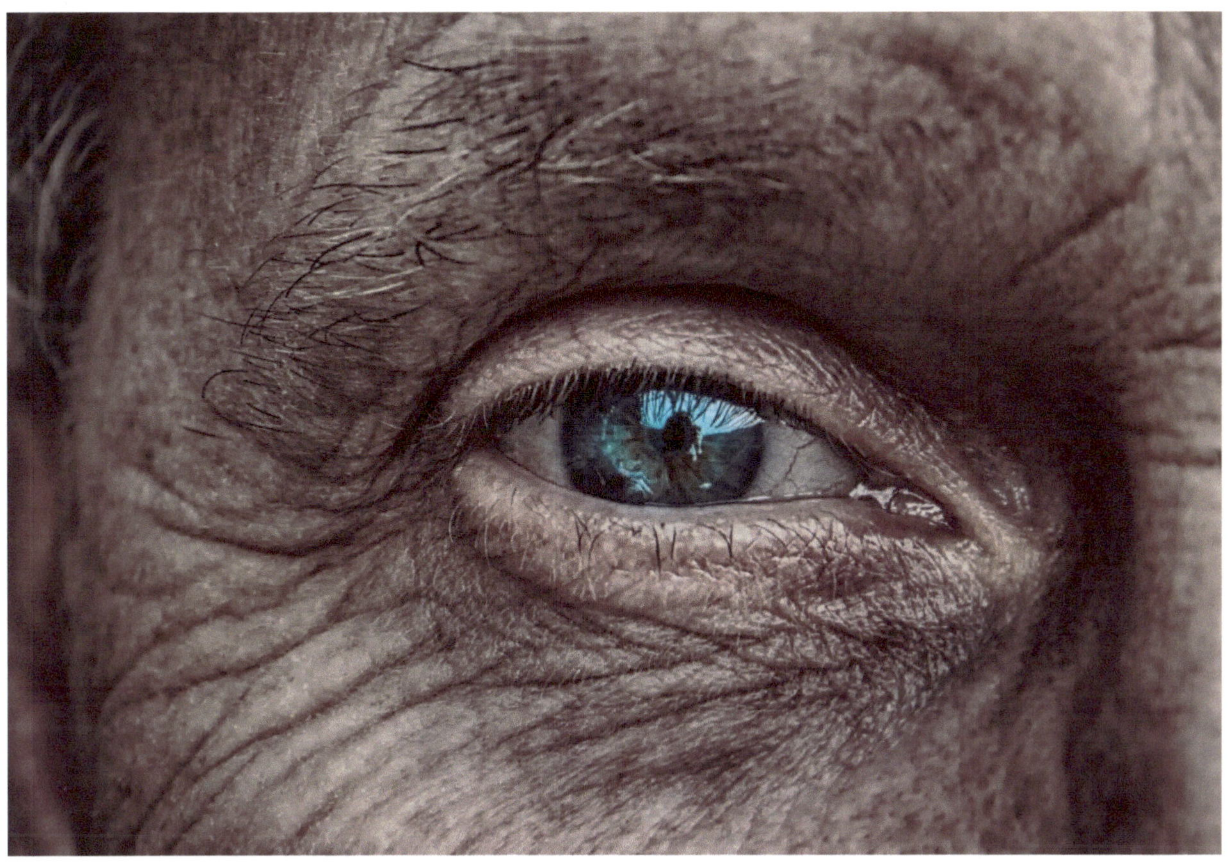

Type One Diabetes (T1D)

T1D only affects around five percent of Americans, and it shares many similarities with T2D, but it develops differently. T1D is an autoimmune disorder, meaning that the immune system attacks and destroys the pancreatic beta cells that produce insulin.

It's unknown why the immune system attacks the pancreatic cells, but during the process, the pancreas stops making insulin, and supplemental insulin is needed from that time on. Symptoms of T1D appear much faster and are much more profound.

Although adults can develop T1D, and men are more at risk than women, it's most prevalent among children, and it typically sets in at puberty. The rate of increase globally is at three percent annually among children.

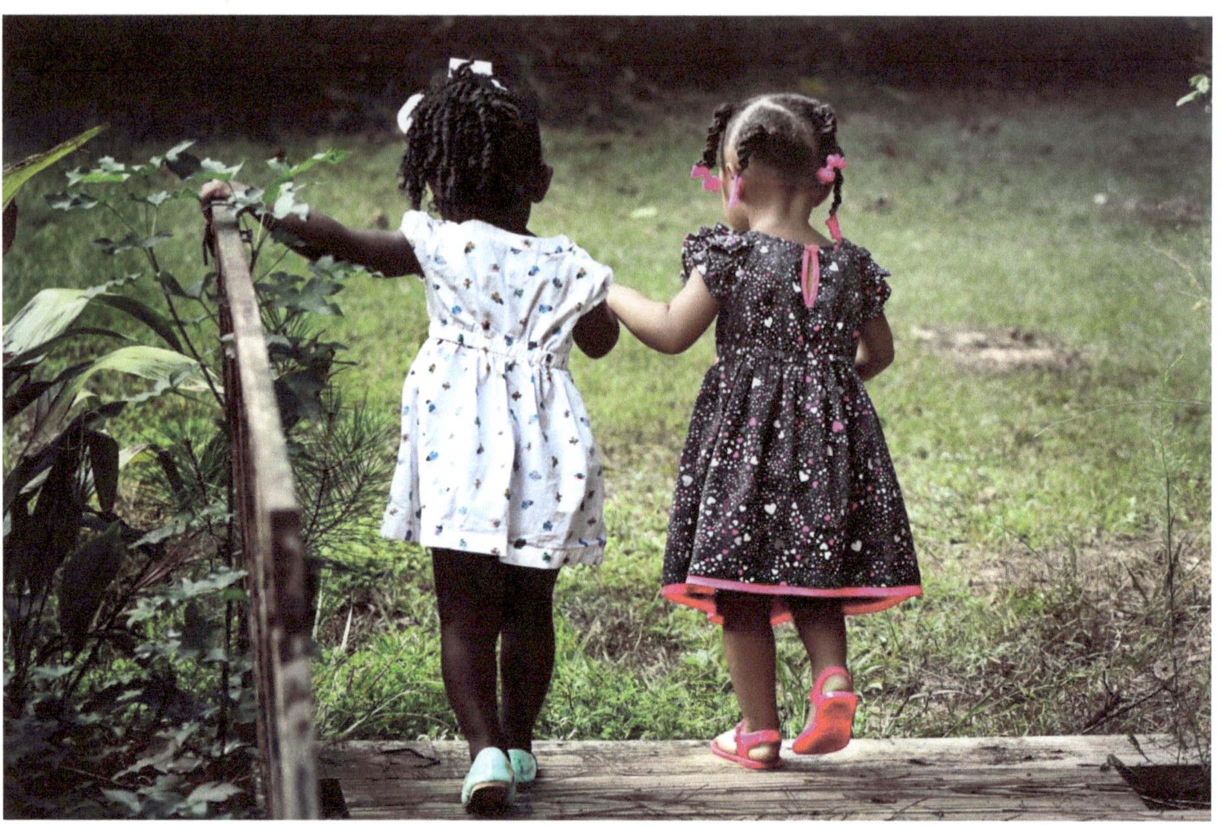

Risk Factors

The risk factors are highly debatable in T1D, but it comes down to a few potential culprits:

- Genetics play a role if a child has beta-cell autoantibodies. This affects the way their bodies process glucose because the antibodies automatically destroy insulin or beta cells.
- According to Stanford Children's Health, being Caucasian increases your risk of developing T1D, which is the opposite of T2D.
- Having cystic fibrosis, which causes scarring on the pancreas that stops the organ from producing insulin, also puts you at higher risk.
- Hemochromatosis, which causes an overload of iron that can damage the beta-pancreatic cells, is also a risk factor.
- Viral childhood infections can also cause T1D, such as rubella, measles, and mumps.
- Many other autoimmune disorders in which the immune system attacks organs such as the pancreas can lead to T1D. Examples of these disorders include celiac disease and thyroid autoimmune disease.
- Stress can lead to autoimmune dysfunction and the subsequent development of T1D.

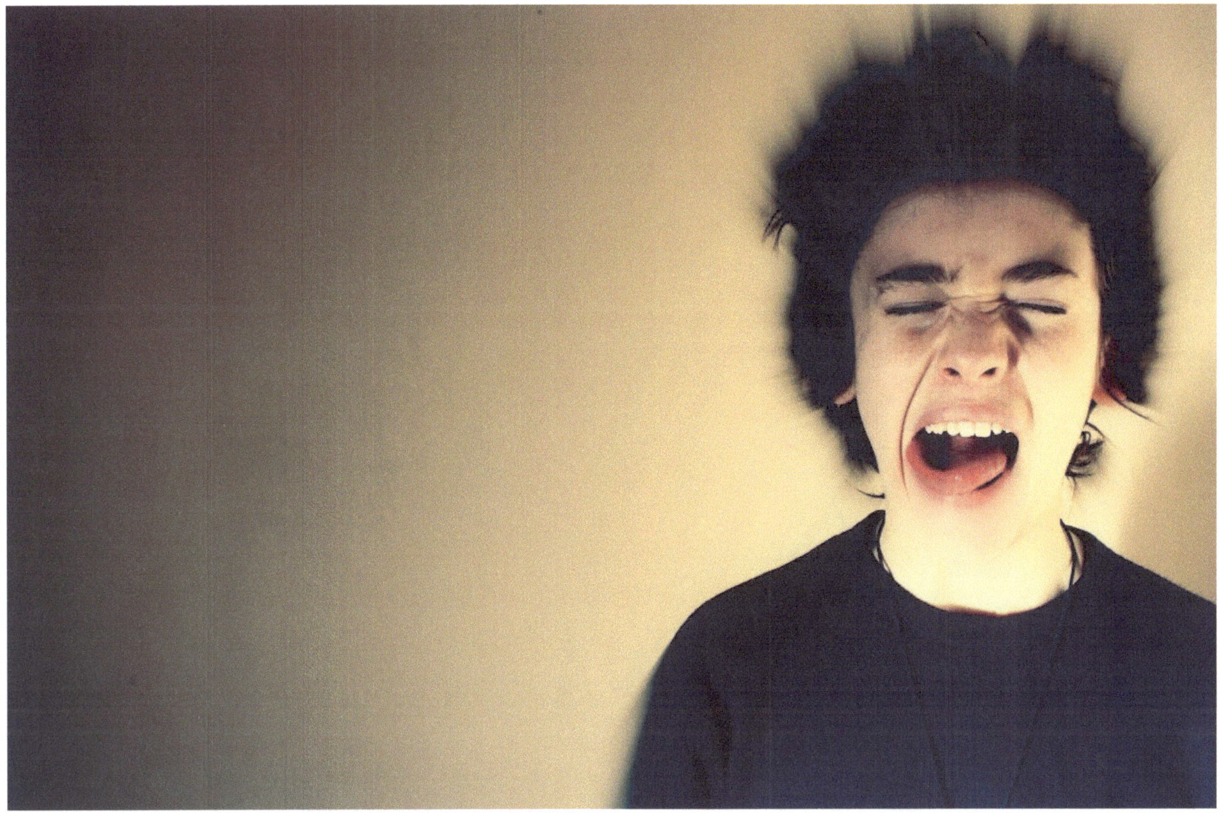

T1D is a challenging condition that affects young and older people, but with proper care, frequent monitoring, and simple lifestyle changes, you can lead a pleasant life with the condition.

Common Symptoms

The symptoms of T2D can manifest in various ways, including:

- Increased urination
- Dehydration and thirst
- Increased appetite
- Blurry vision
- Unexplained fatigue
- Numbness or tingling in the hands and feet
- Wounds that take longer to heal
- Unexpected weight loss
- Thrush

Hyperglycemia is defined as ***high blood glucose levels***. Patients with hyperglycemia exhibit dry mouth, nausea, vomiting, a fruity smell on the breath, difficulty breathing, and coma. Untreated hyperglycemia can be life-threatening.

Hypoglycemia is a potentially life-threatening condition of having ***extremely low blood glucose levels***. Symptoms include shakiness, a pale face, sweating, chills, anxiety, and a rapid heartbeat.

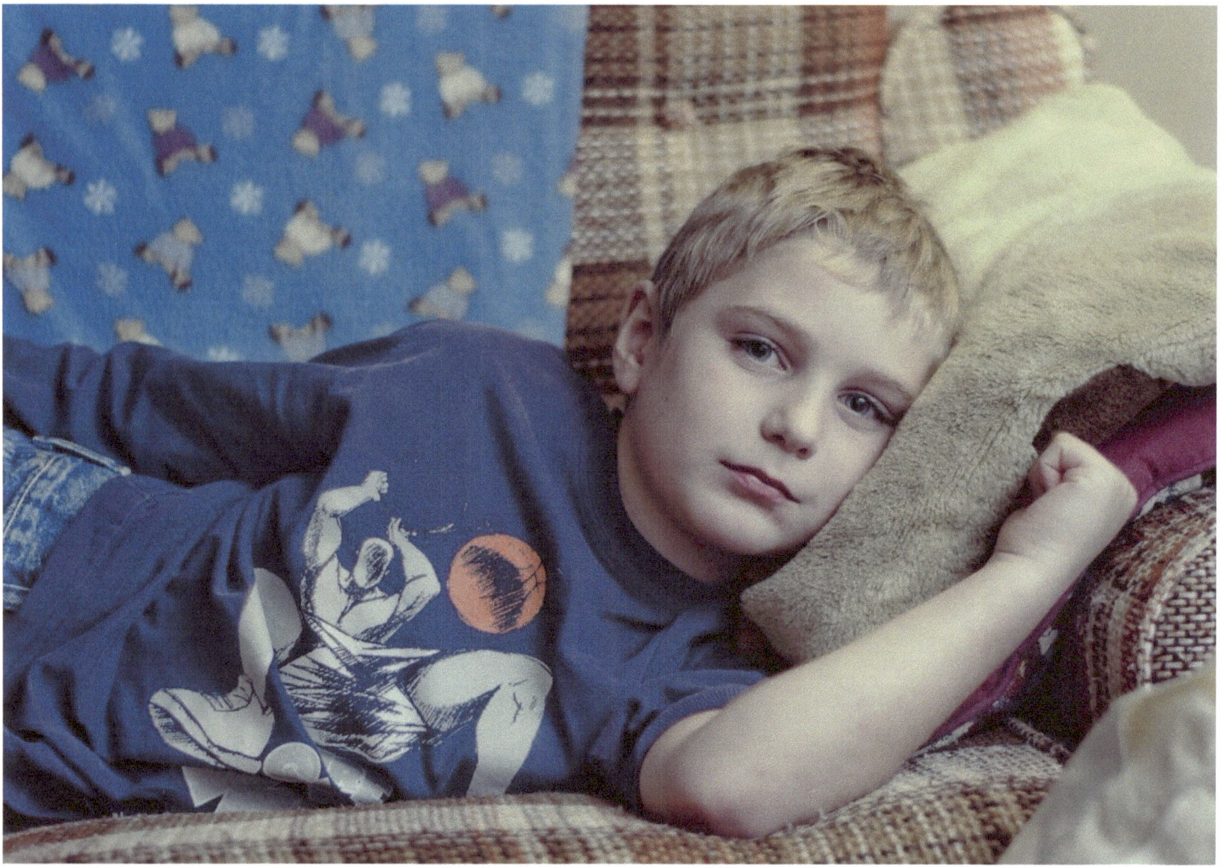

Other hypoglycemic symptoms include dizziness, lightheadedness, nausea, weakness, extreme fatigue, tingling, and severe headaches. If untreated, patients can develop seizures, loss of consciousness, or slip into a coma.

Interestingly enough, the symptoms of hypoglycemia and hyperglycemia occur more commonly in T1D than T2D, and they are more severe in T1D.

Can T2D Change into T1D?

The simple answer is no. Even though the two main types of diabetes share similarities, they aren't caused by the same factors.

Patients who suffer from an uncommon condition called latent autoimmune diabetes in adults (LADA) can be thought to have T2D when they actually have T1D.

LADA mimics T2D, but the fact that it is an autoimmune condition which prevents pancreatic cells from producing insulin makes it a T1D disorder. The LADA test establishes the diagnosis. So, to clarify again, T2D cannot become T1D.

Final Thoughts

Whichever type of diabetes you suffer from, you should adopt a healthier lifestyle to support treatment. Insulin-dependent individuals can't simply throw out their injections. Instead, they should use lifestyle changes to improve their overall health while adequately treating their T1D.

T1D is undoubtedly stressful, but amazing advancements are being made that could change the way we treat it soon. Don't give up hope, even if you must rely on insulin.

Diabetic Complications That Promote Research and Development

Diabetes is a long-term condition that can possibly be reversed in some cases, and in other cases, it can be managed more efficiently to avoid potential complications. Learning about the dangerous complications of diabetes can help you take precautions to prevent these bad outcomes.

The journey to better quality health starts with knowledge.

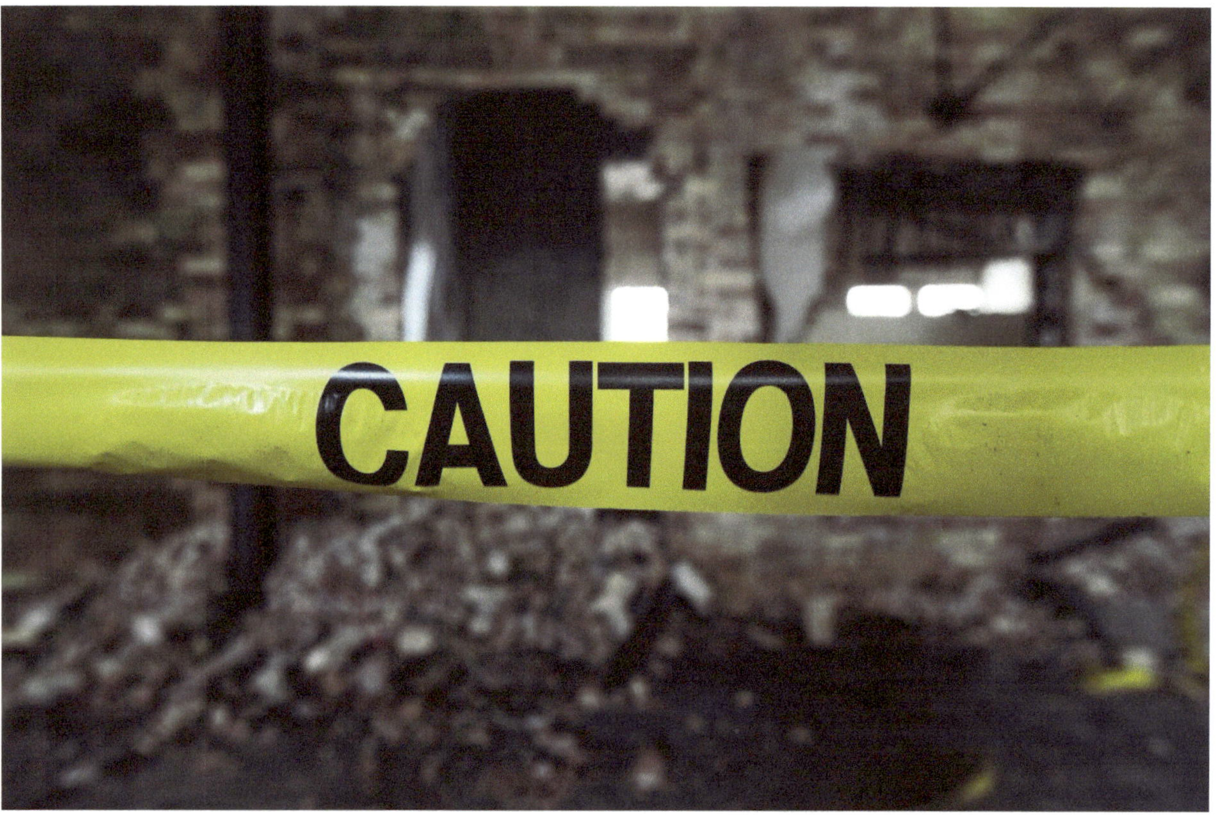

Potential Complications of Inefficient Diabetes Management

Many complications are shared between Type One diabetes (T1D) and Type Two diabetes (T2D), even though they're different conditions. Both conditions can cause increased levels of blood glucose, which is very destructive over time.

Cardiovascular Problems

Persistently high blood glucose levels deteriorate your arteries, leading to cardiovascular problems. The European Cardiology Review published a paper confirming the correlation between T2D and hypertension (high blood pressure).

Arteries become narrowed and hardened, which is called atherosclerosis, and pressure builds in the arteries to keep blood pumping to vital organs. The problem is that over time, the organs become unable to manage blood pressure this high.

Diabetes is also responsible for the increased production of low-density lipoprotein (LDL) cholesterol, which is the bad cholesterol that builds plaque in your arteries, deteriorating them even further and contributing to high blood pressure.

This plaque development in the arteries contributes to the risk of heart disease and hypertension.

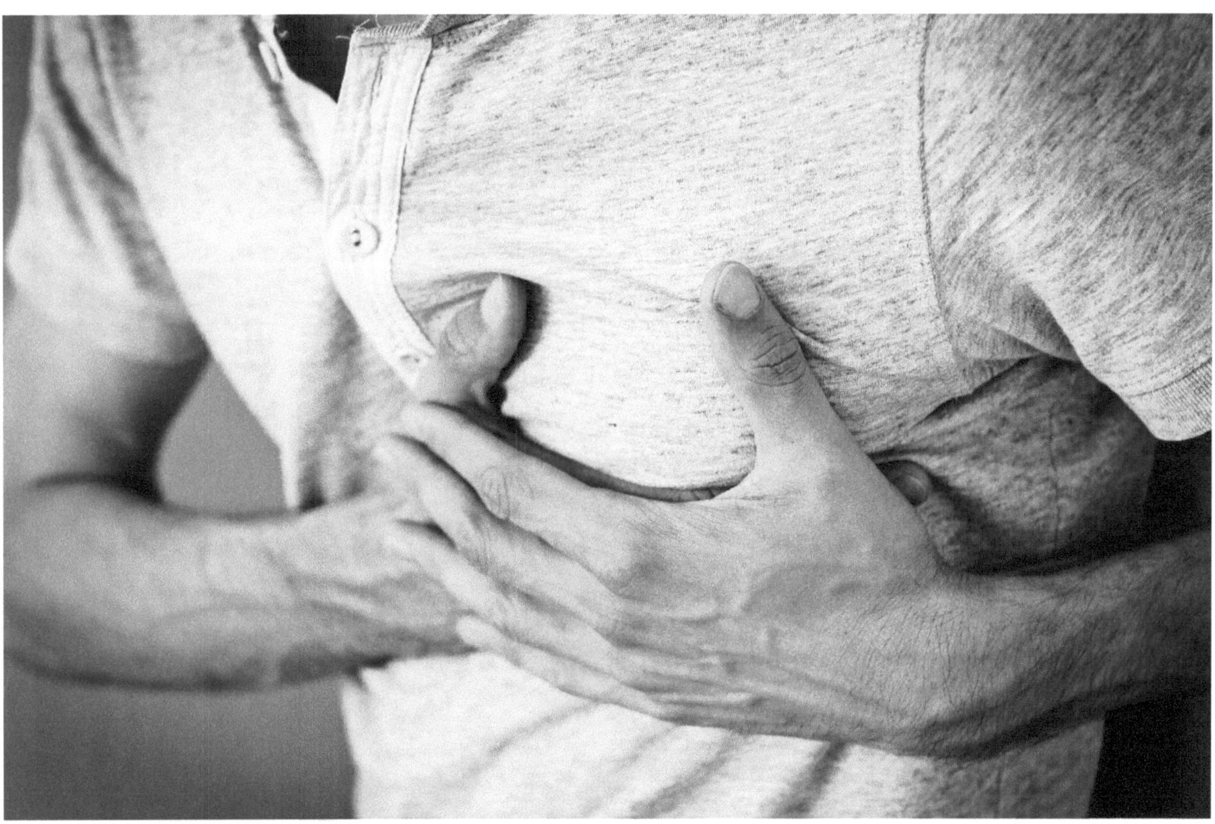

Neuropathy and Other Nerve Damage

The tingling sensations and numbness in your hands and feet are called peripheral neuropathy. Over time, uncontrolled diabetes causes damage to the small capillaries, which supply nerves with nutrients.

The nerves become damaged due to decreased blood supply and nutrients, leading to the condition of neuropathy. It's a very unpleasant complication.

Autonomic nerves connect every organ to the central nervous system (CNS) so that the brain can communicate with the organs and vice versa. These nerves are also subject to damage in patients with uncontrolled diabetes.

Autonomic neuropathy can impact the organs in your body, including the way they function. An example is the complication of an irregular heart rhythm caused by damage to the autonomic nerves connected to the heart.

Chronic Kidney Disease (CKD)

Uncontrolled blood glucose can also damage the small blood vessels in your kidneys, causing CKD when the kidneys can't function and filter waste efficiently anymore.

Gastroparesis

Gastroparesis is a problem where the stomach is malfunctioning. The cause is uncontrolled diabetes, which damages the vagus nerve, the nerve supply to the stomach.

The stomach no longer properly moves food down the digestive tract and stalls your digestion.

Tooth Decay

Tooth decay isn't only ignited by eating refined sugars. It's also increased when the blood vessels intended to provide nutrients to the gums are impaired by high levels of blood glucose.

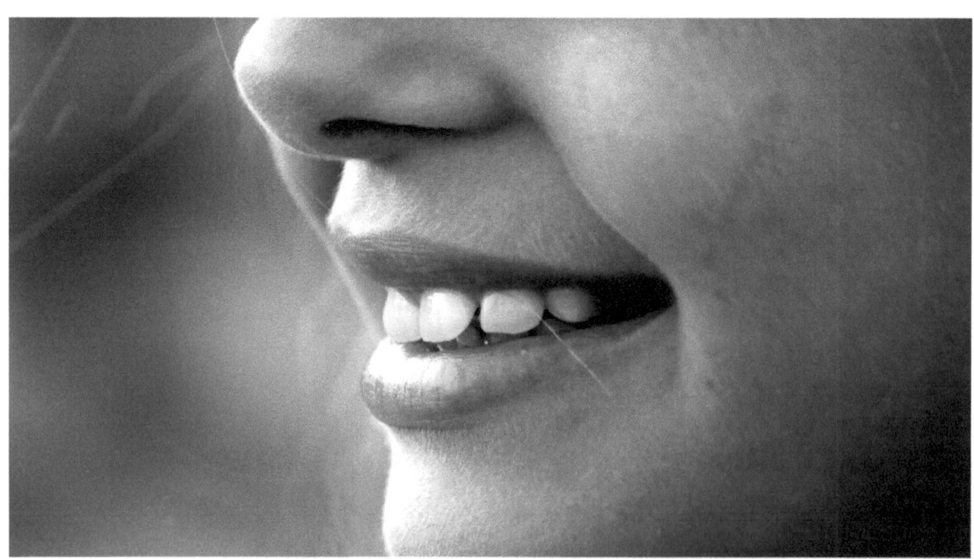

Vision Interference

Diabetes and persistently elevated glucose levels can interfere with or damage your vision. You can suffer from:

- Glaucoma, which happens when pressure builds within your eyes
- Cataracts, which is the clouding of your eye lens
- Diabetic retinopathy, which happens when the blood vessels behind the retina become damaged
- Complete blindness

Stroke

Blood vessel deterioration and associated hypertension from diabetes can increase your risk of stroke. According to the American Diabetes Association (ADA), your risk of having a stroke increases one and half times if you have diabetes.

Foot Ulcers

Mismanaged glucose levels can lead to foot ulcers over time due to decreased circulation and nerve damage. Even worse, injuries to your feet can cause infections that could lead to gangrene and possible amputation.

Depression

It's easy to feel overwhelmed when you must monitor your glucose and ketone levels, and depression often follows overwhelming stress. A lack of knowledge and the constant flow of stress hormones may cause depression in diabetics.

Hearing Loss

Uncontrolled diabetes can lead to trouble hearing, according to the American Speech-Language-Hearing Association (ASHA). Blood vessels and nerve cells are everywhere, including the ears.

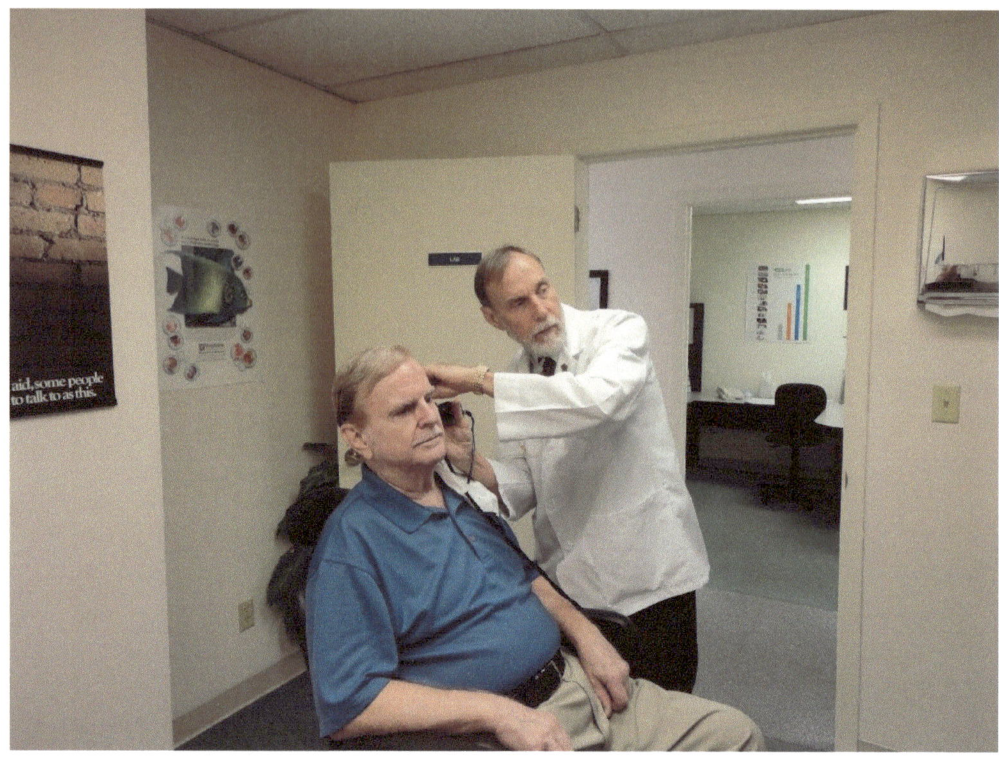

Dementia

Dementia is a degenerative disorder of the brain affecting memory, attention, and cognitive processing. The Alzheimer's Association has seen an increase in the main type of dementia in diabetic patients.

The brain is comprised of multitudes of nerve cells, and high levels of glucose and insulin can damage these cells over time. Insulin can also harm the balance of hormones the brain needs to function properly.

High glucose levels encourage inflammation, which further damages the brain leading to additional difficulties with cognitive function.

Skin and Mouth Problems

Bacterial and fungal infections of the skin and mouth are common if T1D isn't under control.

Pregnancy Complications

Uncontrolled diabetes is a dangerous condition during pregnancy. It can lead to miscarriage, stillbirth, and birth defects.

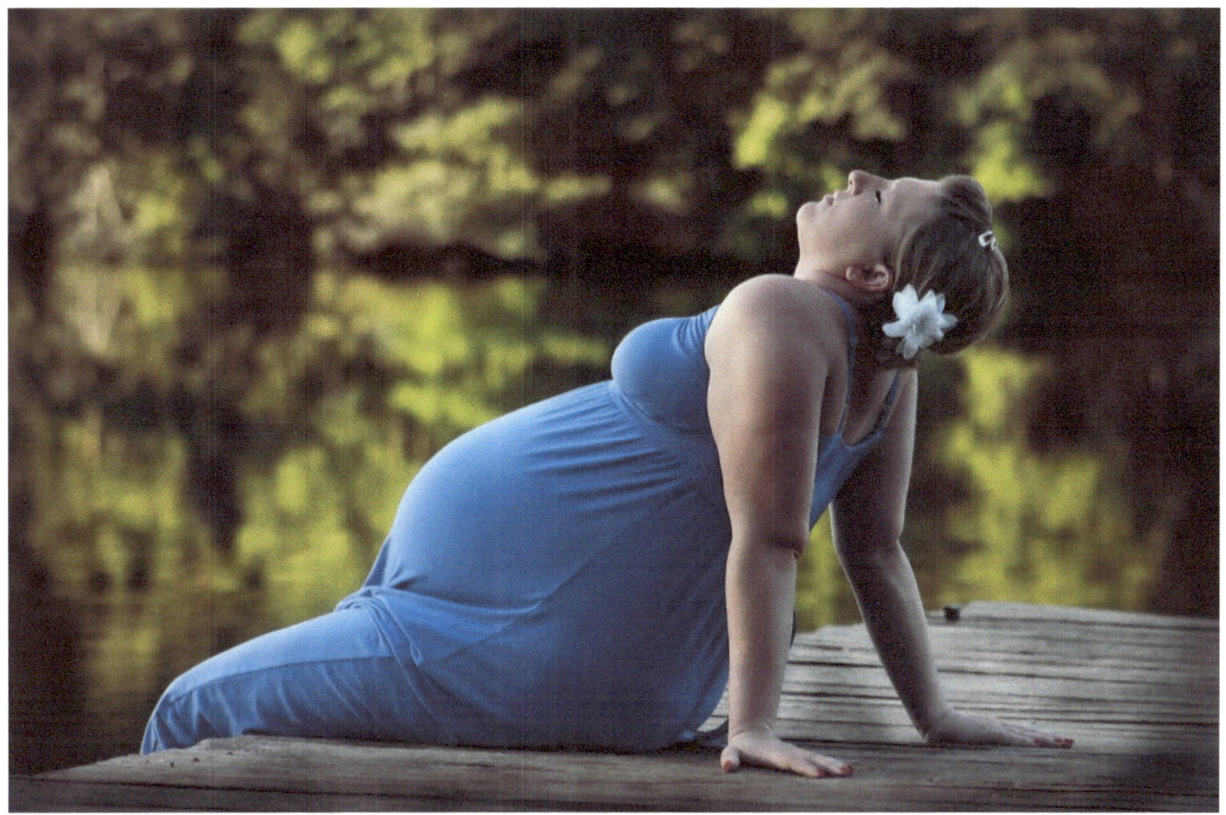

Ketoacidosis

Ketoacidosis is a dangerous shortage of insulin and overproduction of ketones, which are released from fatty acids in the liver when T1D is uncontrolled or undiagnosed. The body turns to fat for energy when there's no insulin left for energy conversion.

Too many ketones can cause acidity in the bloodstream, leading to a life-threatening condition called diabetic ketoacidosis if not treated immediately. T1D people should never willingly induce ketoacidosis.

Final Thoughts

Every condition comes with potential complications, but it's up to you to manage your diabetes carefully. Great advancements are being made to better manage T1D.

T2D patients can rely on supplementing their medication with lifestyle choices and better diets.

Various Traditional Diabetic Medications Offer Pros and Cons

Diabetes is no different from other chronic conditions in that it also requires treatment with medication. Type One (T1D) diabetics must rely on insulin because their bodies cannot produce this glucose regulating hormone.

Type Two (T2D) diabetics often require medications, but they can supplement their traditional drugs with lifestyle changes and autophagy to dramatically improve their condition.

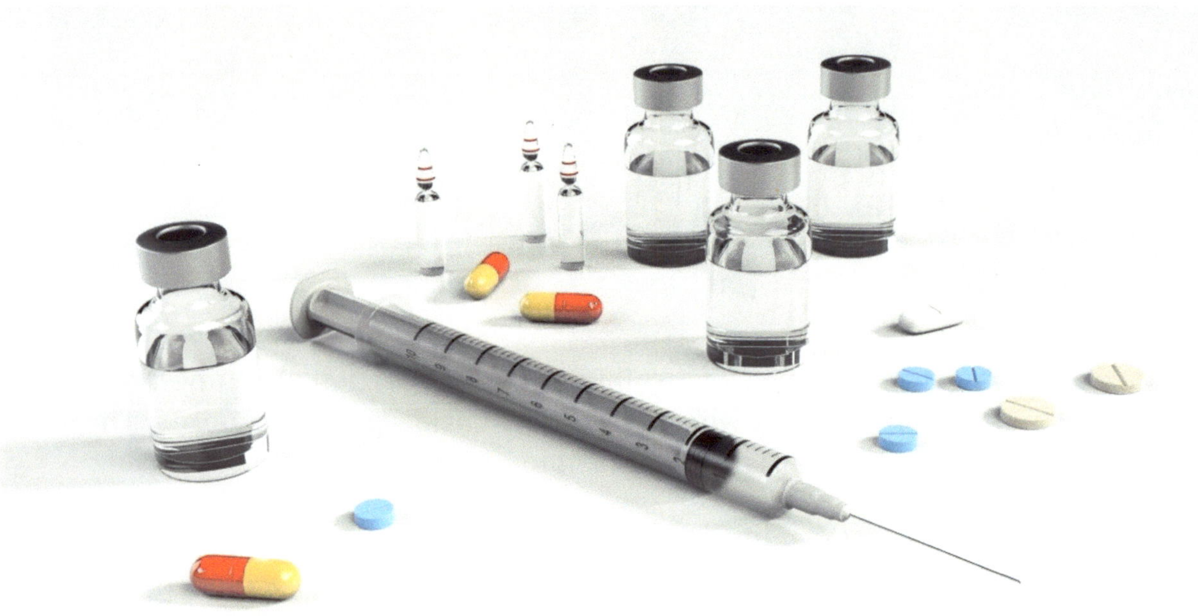

However, understanding what each medication does helps you realize the importance of traditional treatment when it's necessary. Also, knowing the side effects can help guide you to consider alternative treatment, if possible.

Type Two Diabetes Medications

For many, most of the medications they use if they have T2D are oral, but some people also need insulin.

Biguanides

Biguanides are the most common treatment for T2D, and examples are Metformin, Glucophage, and Fortamet.

These drugs decrease the amount of glucose produced by the liver, regulate glucose absorption in the intestines, and increase your sensitivity to insulin.

Biguanides come with potential side effects, such as unintended weight loss, nausea, vomiting, diarrhea, decreased appetite, malaise, and a metallic taste in your mouth. They shouldn't be used if you have kidney or liver problems.

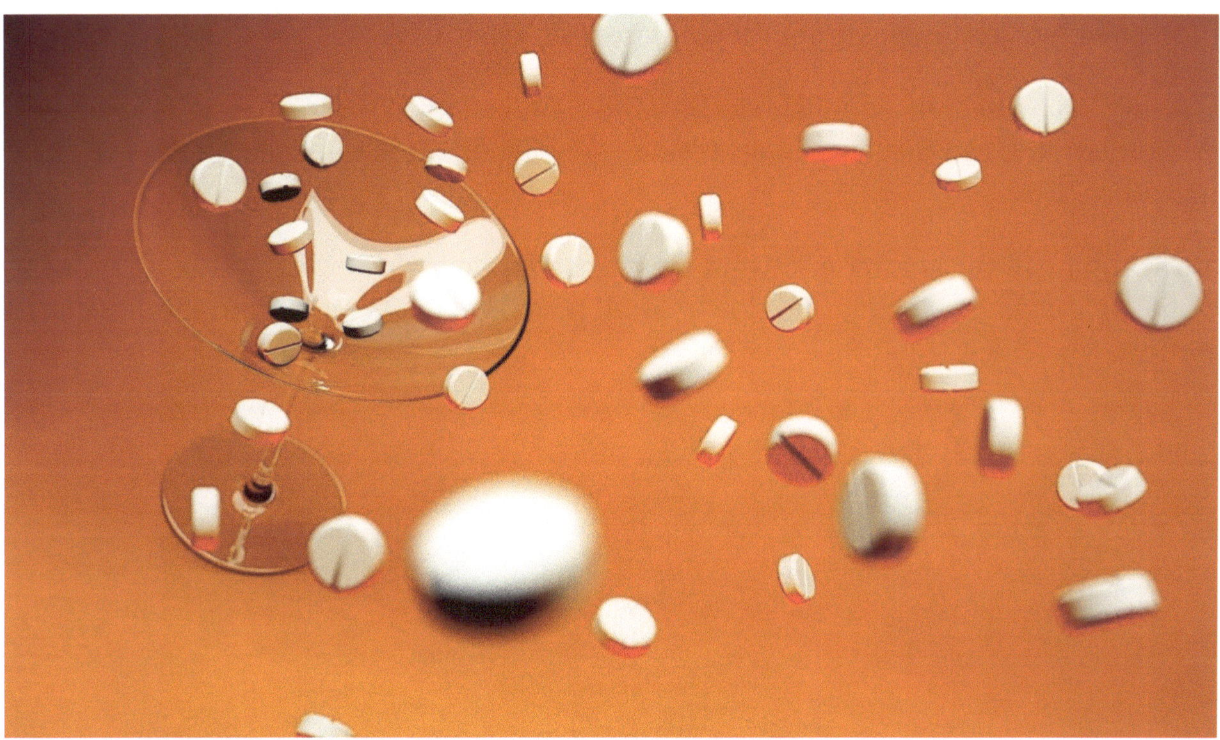

Dipeptidyl Peptidase-4 (DPP-4) Inhibitors

This drug is prescribed along with dietary and lifestyle changes. It includes brand names like Nesina, Canzano, Tradjenta, and Glyxambi. DPP-4 inhibitors are used to produce more insulin when the pancreas has low insulin production.

The potential side effects of DPP-4 inhibitors are migraines, urinary tract infections, and upper respiratory infections, which developed in five percent of patients in a study at Rutgers University.

Sulphonylureas

Sulphonylureas are often supplemental to other diabetic medications, such as Metformin, and some common names are Glimepiride, Glipizide, Glucotrol, and Micronase. These drugs cause the pancreatic beta cells to release more insulin.

The side effects may include weight gain, allergic skin reactions, sensitivity to light, and hypoglycemia, which is low blood sugar.

Thiazolidinediones

Actos is the brand name of this medication, and it acts to decrease glucose production from the liver while enhancing your overall insulin sensitivity.

According to research published by the University of Ioannina in Greece, thiazolidinediones can cause water retention, weight gain, fluid retention in the eyes, and heart failure.

These are some of the common T2D medications and their side effects. If you can make some lifestyle changes, you may be able to avoid these oral medications and the associated side effects.

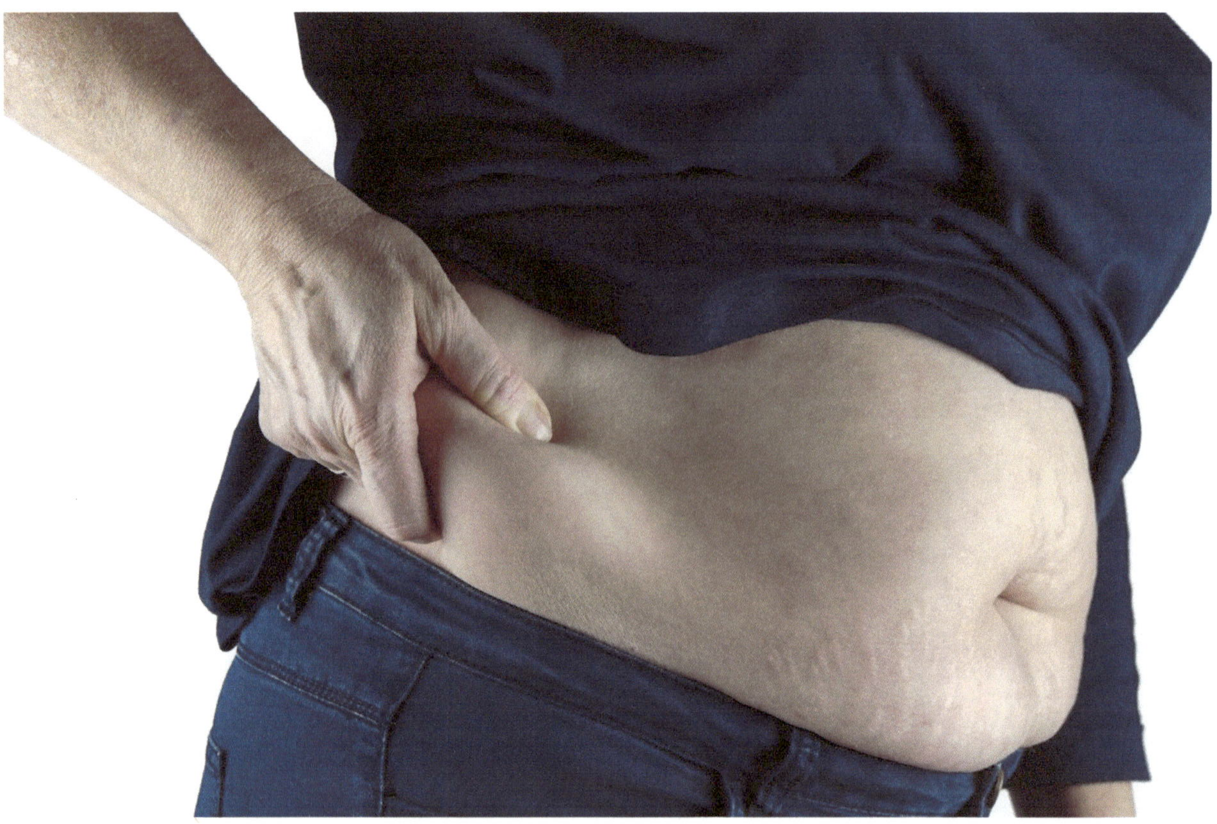

Type One Diabetes Treatment: Insulin

T1D develops when the pancreas can't produce insulin anymore. This shortage of insulin needs to be replenished, and insulin treatment does that very thing.

The type of insulin treatment prescribed depends on your levels of depletion, but it will be one of the following:

Short-Acting Insulin Includes:

- Humulin
- Novolin

Short-acting insulin is a highly effective drug that stimulates the cells to absorb glucose. Some side effects include the possibility of hypoglycemia, allergic reactions, and the development of fatty cells under the injection site.

Intermediate-Acting Insulin Includes:

- Humulin N
- Novolin N

This insulin treatment is similar to the short-acting injections, but it's more convenient. The same side effects may occur, but the advantages of the drug outweigh the cons. You should not use this in pregnancy or if you have chronic kidney disease.

Rapid-Acting Insulin Includes:

- Humalog
- Apidra
- FlexPen
- Fiasp

Rapid-acting insulin treatments carry the same pros and cons as the first two Types.

Long-Acting Insulin Includes:

- Lantus
- Tresiba
- Levemir
- Toujeo

The long-acting insulin treatments are highly effective, and the effects can last for 24 hours or more. It carries similar side effects as the previous types but can also cause hypersensitivity.

Combination Insulins Might Include:

- Novolog Mix
- Humalog Mix
- Ryzodeg

The combination insulin treatments are also very effective, and they come with some similar side effects. The specific combination will need to be tailored to the individual patient. If you have kidney or liver problems, you likely should not be using this treatment, but check with your doctor.

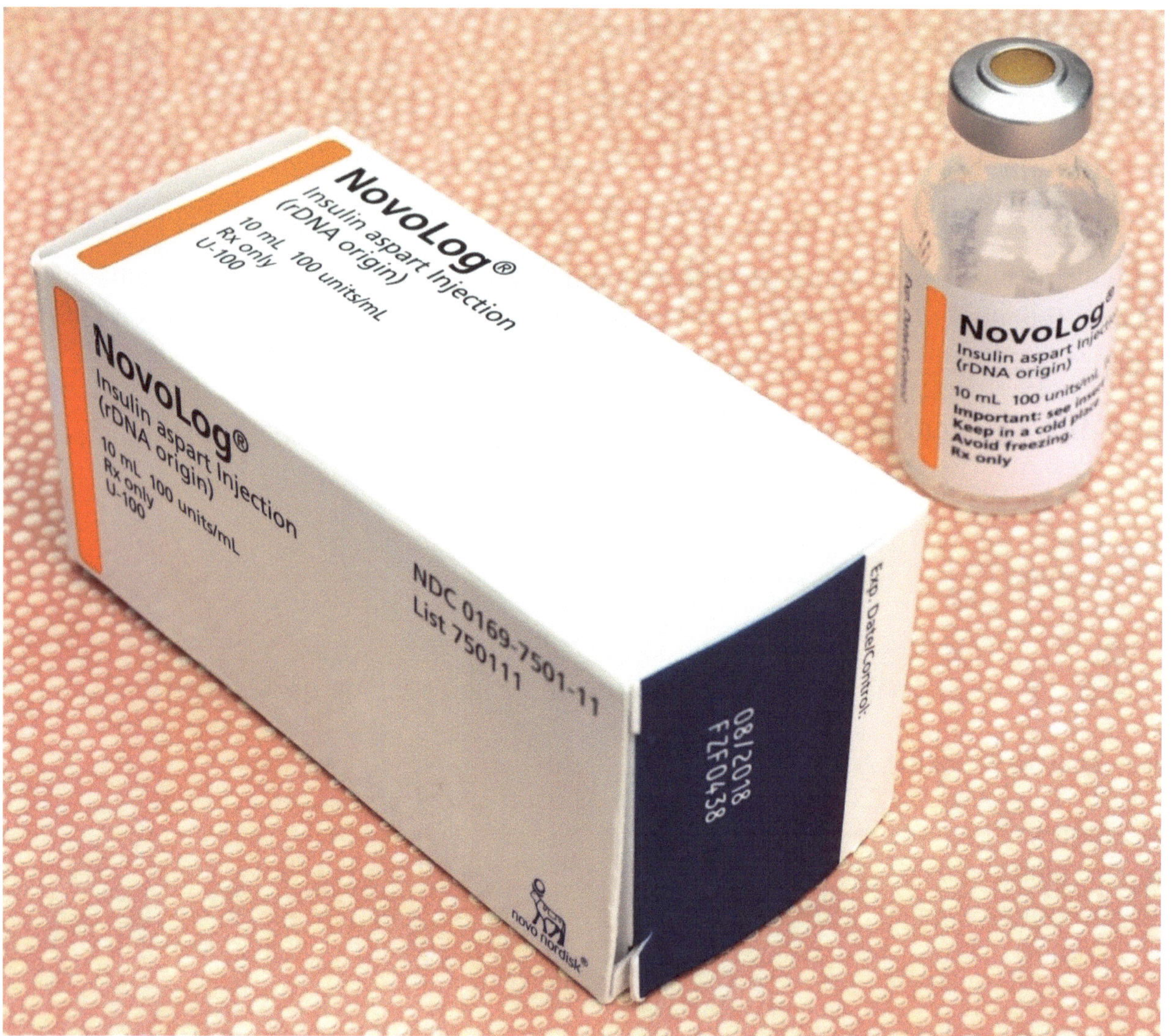

Amylinomimetic Injections

Another injectable drug prescribed to people with T1D is called Amylinomimetic, Pramlintide, or SymLinPen, which is injected before meals to help you digest food and keep your glucose levels low by inhibiting its production.

The main disadvantage of using insulin or injectable treatments is that you'll have to build a tolerance for needles, which can't be avoided.

Insulin Pumps

Insulin pumps are tiny computer devices that act as an artificial pancreas and pump short-acting insulin consistently. They even regulate different doses as you eat. Pumps are highly effective if you monitor your glucose and ketone levels.

An insulin pump should be used with very close supervision by your physician. Some disadvantages include the risk of infection at the site, pump malfunctions, and ketoacidosis, which is a serious diabetic complication.

However, the insulin pump is one of many biotechnical advancements in T1D.

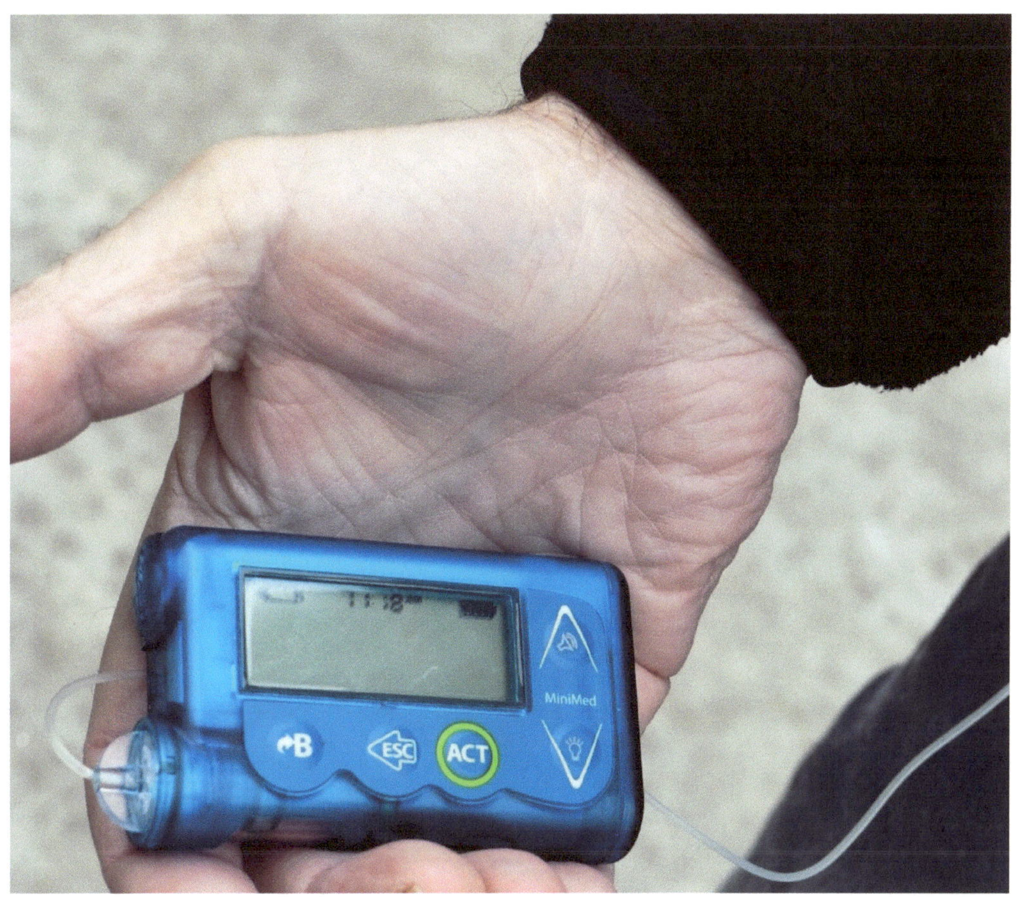

Final Thoughts

Whether you're taking oral medication or injections of insulin, diabetes medical treatments have developed to improve glucose management. Close medical supervision is the key to success in treatment.

The Biotechnical Race Attempting to Cure Diabetes - Part One

Diabetes has become a global epidemic, affecting 422 million people, an increase from 100 million from just 24 years ago. With this trajectory, it's become clear that developing a cure is a high priority.

The biotech industry is making tremendous strides, especially for Type One diabetes (T1D). But Type Two diabetes (T2D) is also concerning because it comes with many potential complications if poorly managed.

Recent advancements in the industry have improved the ability to monitor this condition much better, and other research is very promising for the future.

Let's look at these exciting advancements.

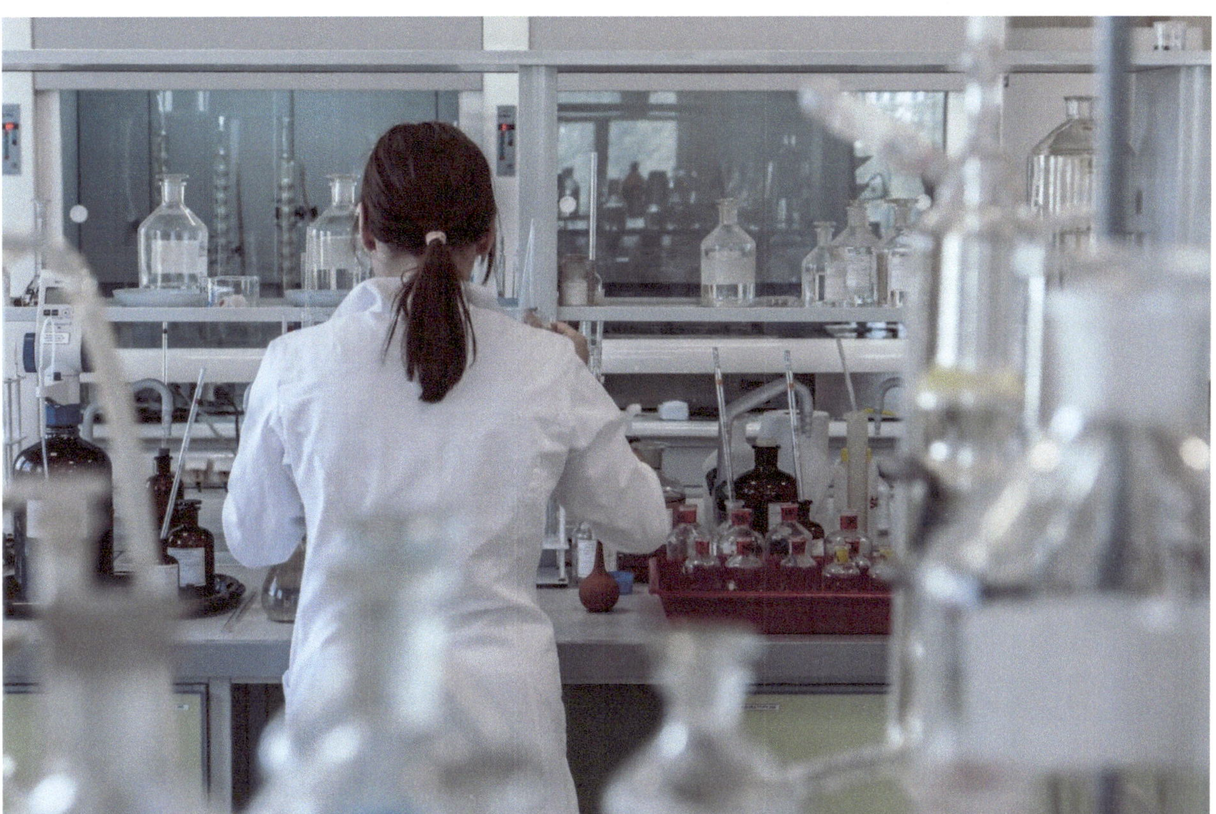

Diabetic Monitoring Advancements

As science and technology stride forward in the war against diabetes, glucose monitoring continues to improve.

The first product being developed is called the smart contact lens. Jihun Park and his colleagues at the Ulsan National Institute of Science and Technology in South Korea have already created a prototype.

The lens looks like a regular contact lens, and it's designed for comfort. As soon as your glucose levels spike, the lens switches over to light-emitting diode (LED) mode, which allows you to read your glucose levels in a mirror.

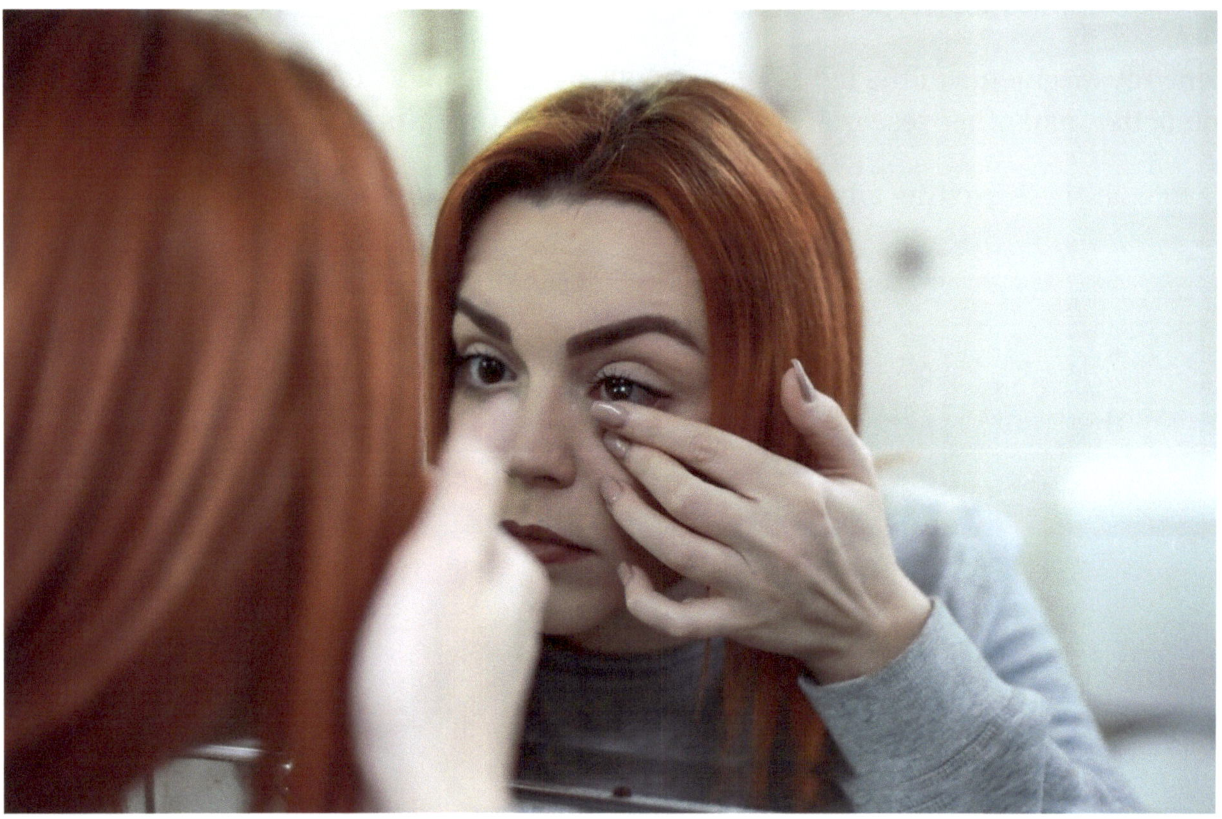

Another non-invasive monitoring method is adding special ink to tattoos. Created at the Massachusetts Institute of Technology (MIT) and Harvard, the color-changing ink turns brown when your glucose levels spike.

The pleasant point about these ideas is that they offer ways to monitor your glucose levels without pricking your fingers. Another non-invasive monitor includes a graphene patch that monitors hair follicles.

The needle-free monitoring revolution has begun, but challenges still need to be overcome.

Lexicon Inhibitor Trials

Another therapeutic approach is under investigation in T1D, and more research might make this a viable option for T2D. Lexicon Pharmaceuticals has run successful trials of a new drug called LX4211.

This drug targets the sodium-glucose transporter 1 (SGLT1) in the digestive tract, which absorbs glucose from the bloodstream. It also targets the SGLT cells surrounding the kidneys, which are responsible for reabsorbing glucose.

This scientific trial studied patients with T1D taking a 400mg dose of the drug over a 30-day period. The drug was effective in allowing the patients to excrete the excess glucose by the kidneys.

Previously, this drug had shown the ability to increase certain hormones that improve glycemic index and appetite in patients. The plan is to expand the trials and examine how successful this drug can be in T2D as well.

Targeted Immunotherapy

Immunotherapy is another advancement in treating T1D. Recall that T1D is caused by the autoimmune phenomenon where the immune cells attack insulin-producing cells. Belgian biotech Imcyse had some success in phase one of their trials with immunotherapy.

It's estimated that newly diagnosed T1D patients still have up to 10% of their original beta cells for three to six months after the T1D diagnosis is first made. Imcyse took 41 recently diagnosed patients and conducted a trial on targeted immune cell eradication.

The trial lasted six months, and the drug proved effective in eliminating the autoimmune cells responsible for destroying the beta cells in the pancreas.

This result has been a great success, but a key requirement for the immunotherapy to work is that patients get started with therapy as soon as possible after diagnosis. Otherwise, the pancreatic beta cells will already be destroyed by the disease.

Diabetic Vaccines

Professor Bart Roep from the Department of Diabetes Immunology is working on a vaccine intended to correct the immune system in T1D patients before it destroys too many pancreatic B cells to prevent the onset of T1D.

With this method, you are attempting to stop the autoimmune problem before it even begins. In the process, blood is taken from the patient, and white blood cells are isolated to create dendritic cells.

Dendritic cells train other immune cells like T-cells to recognize that pancreatic beta cells are not real pathogens and shouldn't be attacked.

The dendritic cells are then grown in a lab for six days in a solution with vitamin D so that they become anti-inflammatory, which improves their function.

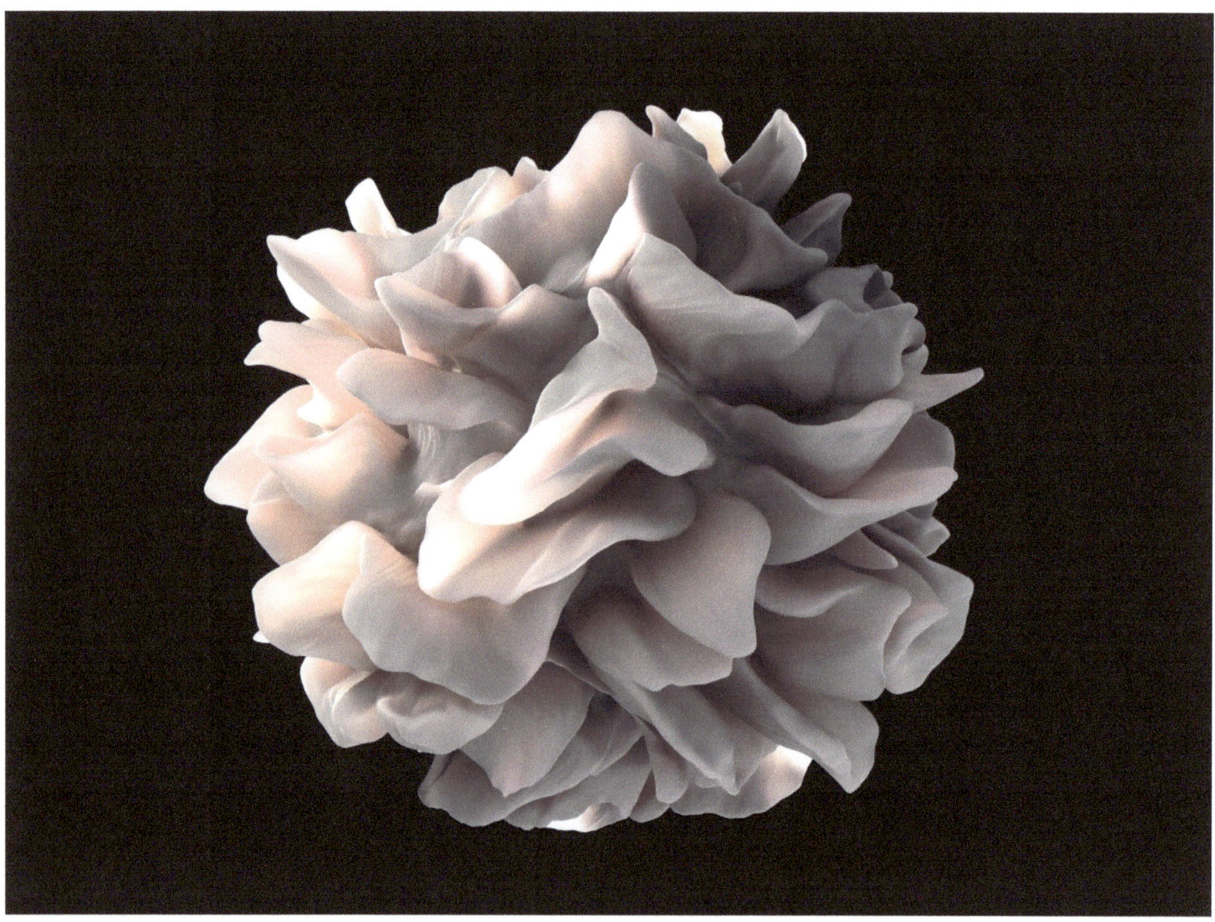

Then they are treated in a proinsulin solution to build a tolerance. Proinsulin is an autoantigen protein that normally destroys beta cells.

This is how the training takes place before you receive the vaccine; the dendritic cells train the T-cells not to destroy the insulin-producing cells, and these trained cells then become regulatory T-cells, which prevent other immune cells from attacking your pancreas.

The vaccine is administered by a patch, which is placed on the abdomen where your pancreas lies. The patch has many microneedles that inject the trained immune cells into the body, where they make their way into the pancreas.

The first study was conducted on nine patients with T1D who continued their insulin treatments for six months while also using the patches. The results showed no further damage to the pancreatic beta cells. These are very promising results warranting further study.

Final Thoughts

The work being done in science and technology is bringing us closer to a cure for diabetes. From non-invasive monitoring to vaccines, we're taking steps closer. There is hope to find more advancements in this debilitating disease.

The Biotechnical Race Attempting to Cure Diabetes - Part Two

Some advancements in research have potentially brought us closer to the goal of finding a cure or better method of treating Type One (T1D) and Type Two diabetes (T2D).

Both conditions can lead to serious complications. Let's see what further developments are undergoing research now.

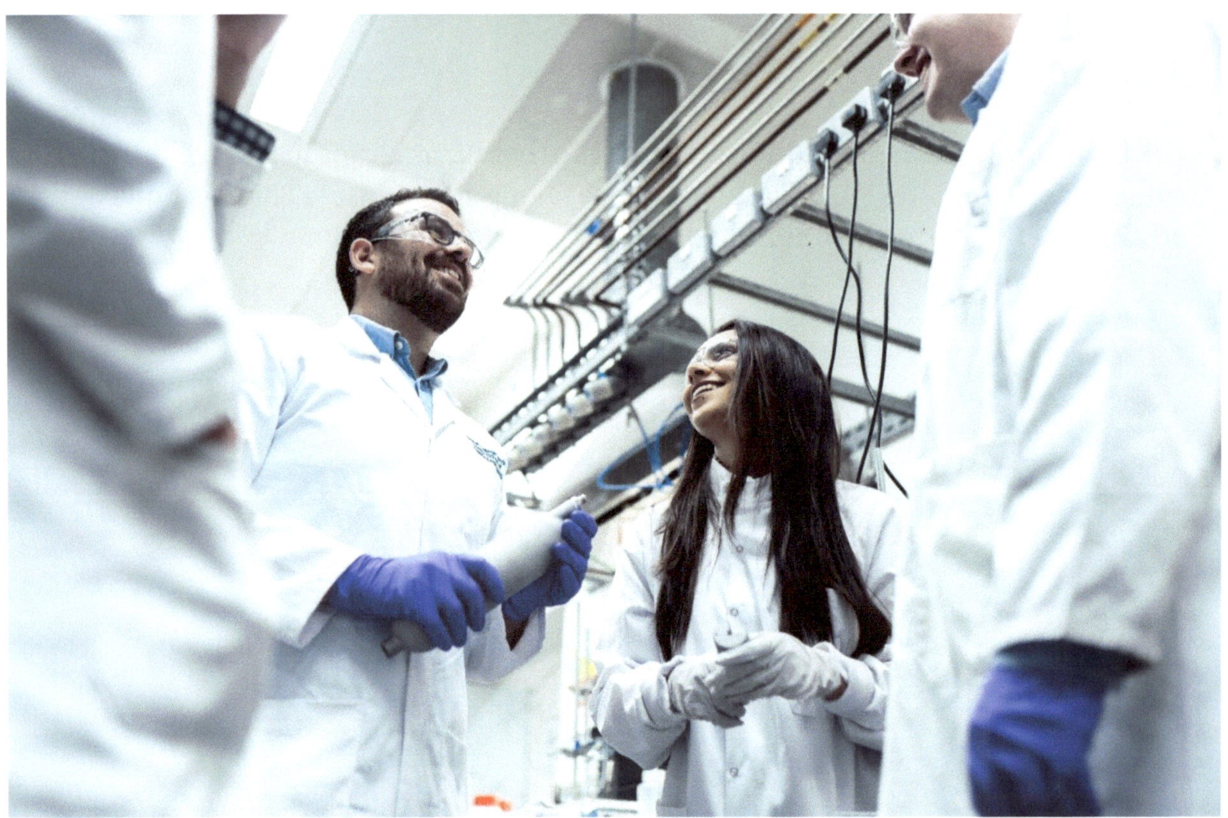

The Mexican Cavefish

What does a fish have to do with diabetes? This chubby, blind cave-dweller has evolved to be insulin resistant. Intrigue abounds when comparing the cave-dweller to its river-dwelling counterpart from the same species.

Insulin is released from the pancreatic B cells after eating, and this regulatory hormone latches onto receptors in your muscles, liver, and fat. Insulin absorbs the glucose from carbohydrates in the bloodstream into the cells.

Your blood glucose levels normalize, and some glucose is burned for energy while some is stored as glycogen for later use. When your body starves, the pancreas releases glucagon, which converts glycogen back to glucose for energy.

Biologist Misty Riddle from the Stowers Institute for Medical Research examined the cave-dwelling fish closely to understand how it survived in its environment if it was insulin resistant.

The cave-dwellers glucose levels were up and down after eating and fasting for 21-days, much more so than the river-dwelling fish. The cave-dwelling fish converted their proline amino acids to leucine amino acids, a phenomenon seen in cases of severe insulin resistance.

These fish have evolved to be diabetic, but they're also living longer than the river-dwelling fish, confirming that they've adopted alternative mechanisms to thrive even in their diabetic state.

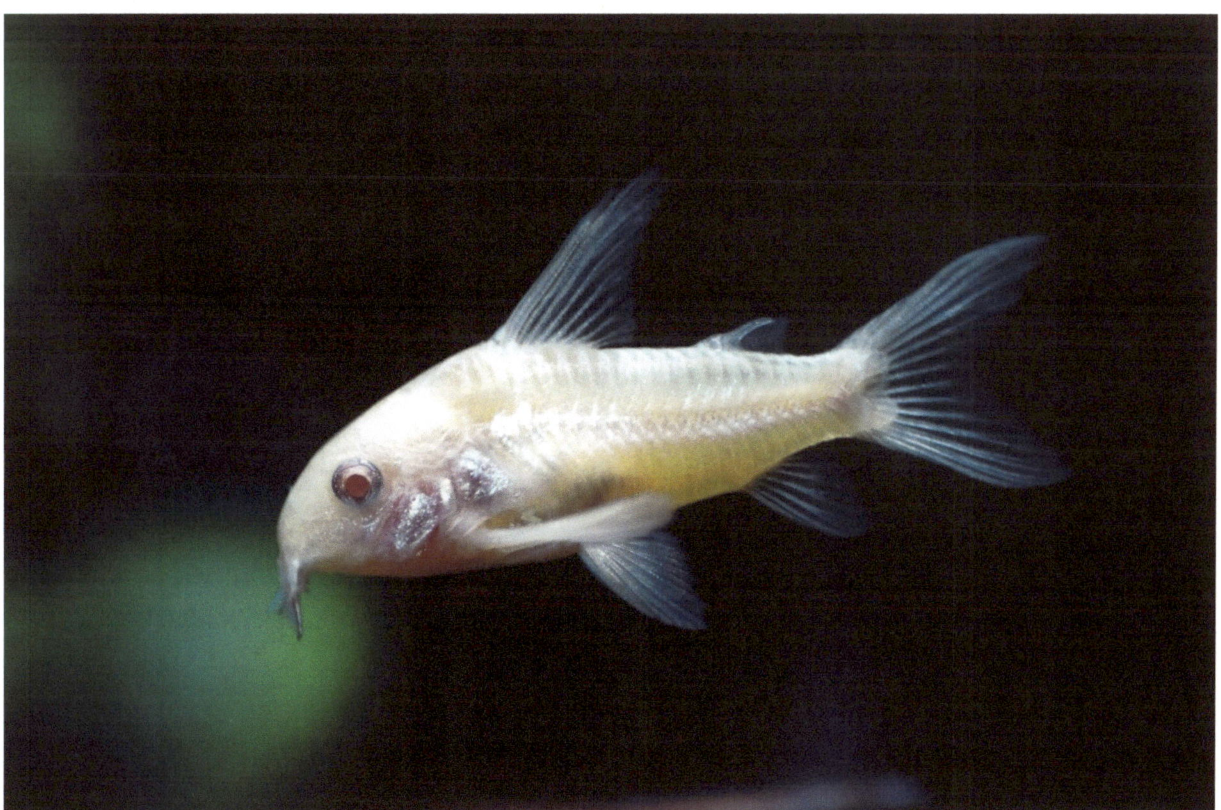

The Mexican cavefish phenomenon provides a means to investigate how T2D patients could adapt their natural homeostasis and avoid complications of their underlying diabetes.

The Microbiome

The microbiome is the collection of bacteria that protects your stomach, and it has a role in hormone regulation and the immune system. Imbalances in this gut flora can be a source of problems in managing diabetes.

Trials are currently underway to enhance the flora and add a variety of bacteria that could help diabetics restore gut flora imbalances.

Virgin Beta Cells

Islet transplant therapy is when clusters of pancreatic cells from donors are transplanted into diabetic patients so that they can produce insulin again.

During recent research, astonishing evidence was found of a new type of cell in the pancreatic islets clusters, which are the cells attacked and depleted in T1D.

Among the clusters were immature beta cells, also called "virgin beta cells." The question was whether these previously unnoticed cells could be matured to function as insulin-producing cells.

Mark Huising from the University of California and his colleagues are currently researching the virgin cells to determine whether they can be matured to respond to glucose levels in the bloodstream and release the necessary insulin.

The immature beta cells lack the receptors to determine blood glucose levels. Further research will be needed to determine if these cells can subsequently develop these receptors and become fully functional.

Artificial Pancreas

A few different types of artificial pancreas exist today. Insulin pumps and the apps that work with them help parents monitor and care for children with T1D. The apps monitor glucose levels, and the pump automatically injects the right dose.

The concept of the artificial pancreas is to replace the organ with newly placed virgin beta cells that are manipulated to prevent the immune system from attacking them.

Researchers are still faced with two of the biggest problems: The scarcity of donors making it hard to conduct human trials and overcoming the immune system response to the virgin beta cells.

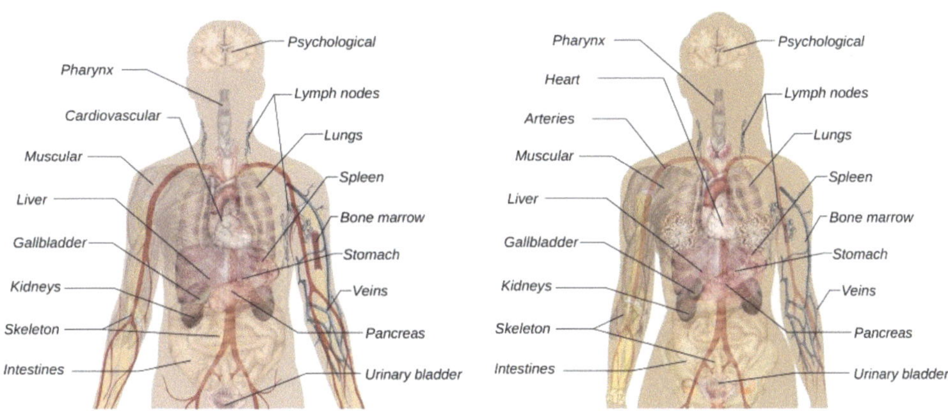

However, a new bioengineered pancreas was tested in a different body location, and the results from one woman's improved T1D showed some success. The female T1D patient had the artificial organ transplanted into her omentum, and she had improvement of her T1D.

The omentum is a large, flat tissue made of a fatty membrane in front of the intestines. The artificial organ in that region mimicked the pancreas more successfully than other transplant sites.

Improvement in three areas will be beneficial in the advancement of the artificial pancreas:

1. Faster-acting insulin.
2. The use of Amylin, another hormone that improves the activity of insulin.
3. Improving insulin dose algorithms.

Great strides have been made so far but overcoming these problems will be a considerable advance in the treatment and methodology of curing T1D.

Final Thoughts

Learning from nature always helps science advance in treating chronic conditions, and the success of various therapy trials continues to grow.

There might not be a cure for diabetes today, but the future holds promise for millions of people globally that it can be better controlled and managed.

Effective Diabetic Treatments to Supplement Your Strategy

Understanding the type of diabetes you have is part one of this journey. However, research in the pursuit of a cure for Type One (T1D) and Type Two diabetes (T2D) has unveiled more interesting treatment supplementation options.

No one deserves to suffer from the potential complications of this debilitating condition, and using the correct medications assisted by expert homecare and lifestyle changes can make a huge difference.

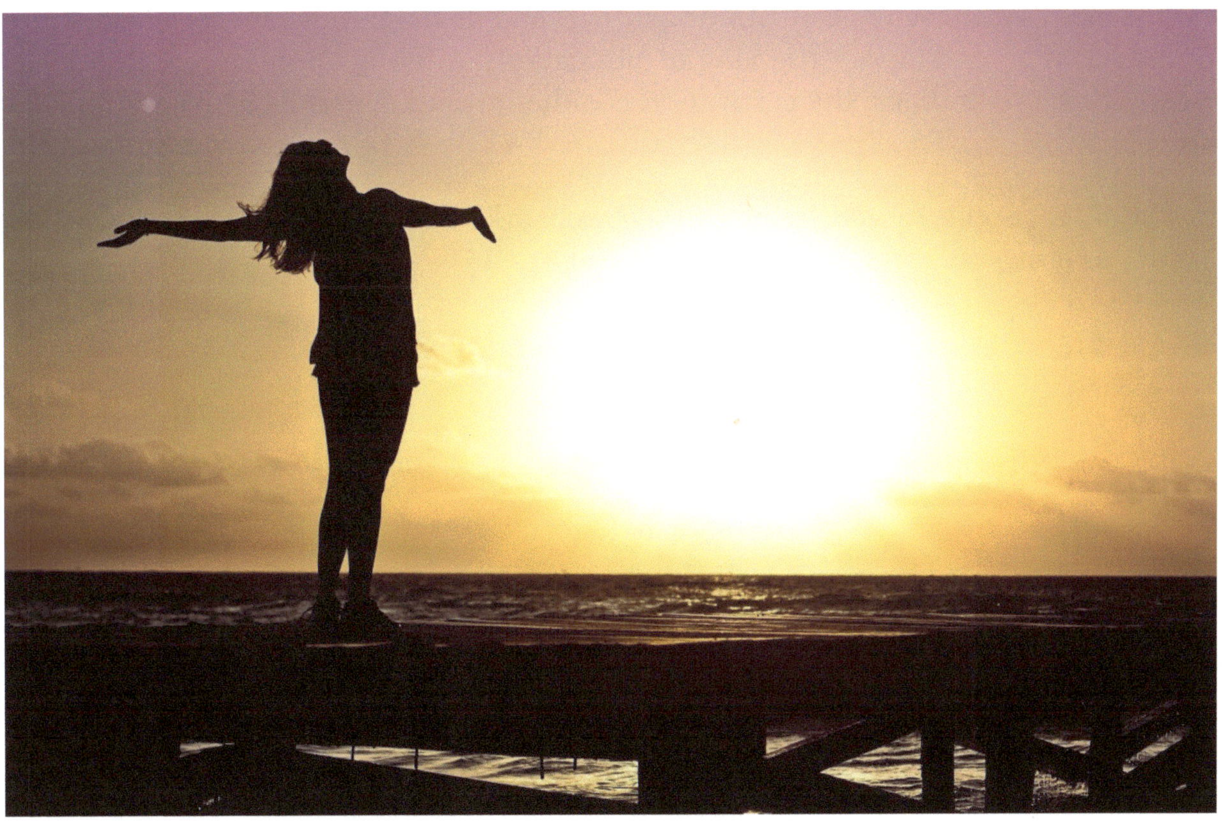

Friends Are Beneficial

Often, taking care of your condition at home with expert guidance is enough to elude the consequences of T2D. However, isolation and loneliness can impact your progress when you're trying to manage diabetes.

A study published in the *BMC Journal* in 2017, called "the Maastricht study," provided a new outlook on socializing and diabetes. With nearly 3,000 participants between 40 and 75, the study showed a correlation between diabetes and loneliness.

Social activity was collected from all participants through self-report questionnaires. A third of the participants were either diagnosed with T2D before or during the experiment.

The study found that male and female participants with smaller social networks were more likely to suffer from T2D.

Additionally, the proximity of the social network, including friends and relatives, was another determining factor for women with T2D, while men with housemates were less likely to have T2D.

The three main social factors contributing to T2D and its magnitude are social isolation, no friends close by, and too few friends and interactions. Although no clear scientific basis is known for these findings, the correlation is quite intriguing and likely has significant value.

High-risk T2D people should broaden their networks and increase social interaction frequency as it may improve diabetes management.

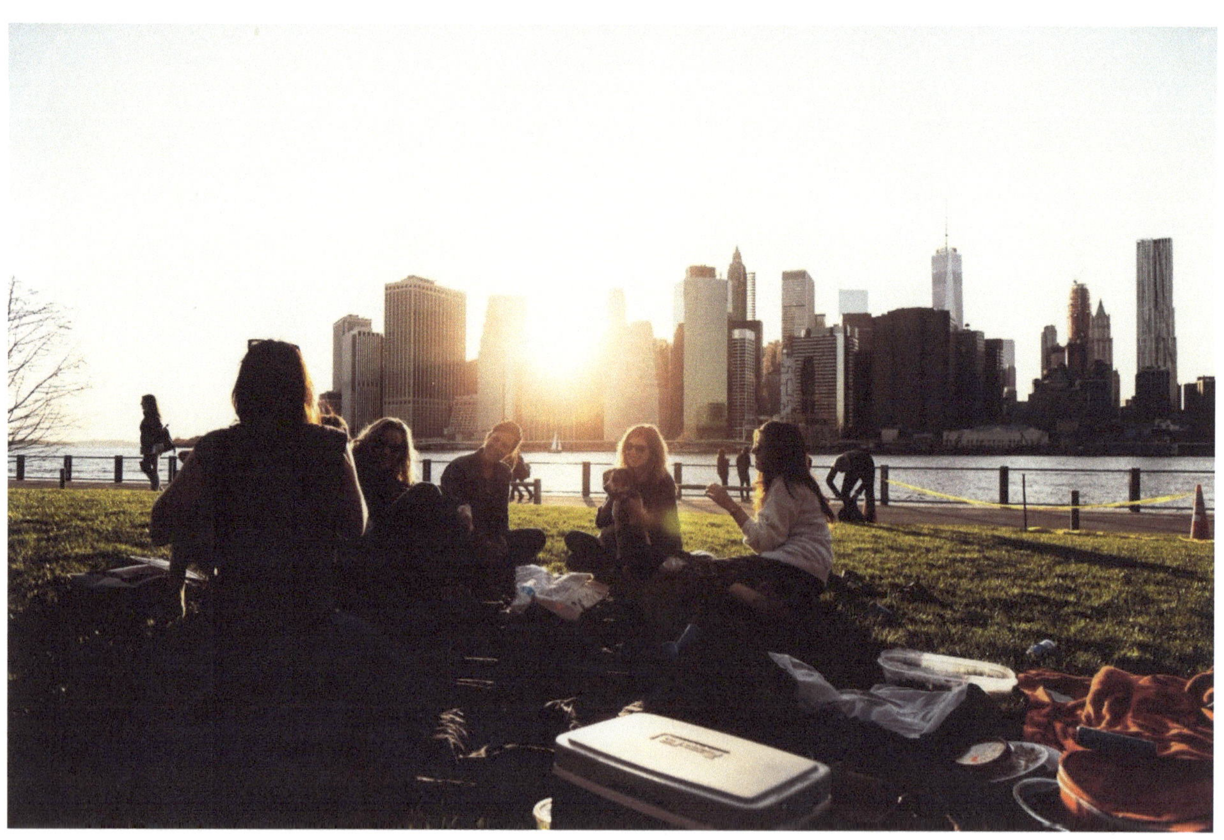

A Common Supplementation

People with T1D should also follow expert advice to care for themselves at home; however, they might have another interesting advantage with a different medication.

The University of Colorado Anschutz Medical Campus found that a common drug listed on the World Health Organization's (WHO) essential drugs list also doubles as a diabetic supplement for people at risk of T1D or the progression of its early stage.

A blood pressure drug called Methyldopa has proven to block the human leukocyte antigen serotype group eight (HLA-DQ8) molecule, which is responsible for attacking your beta cells in the development of T1D.

About 60% of people who have a risk of developing T1D possess this molecule.

A supercomputer was used to run algorithms to determine the efficacy of the Methyldopa, and not only did it prevent the molecule from destroying beta cells, but it also didn't impair other immune cells.

The university researched the drug over ten years on mice and T1D patients.

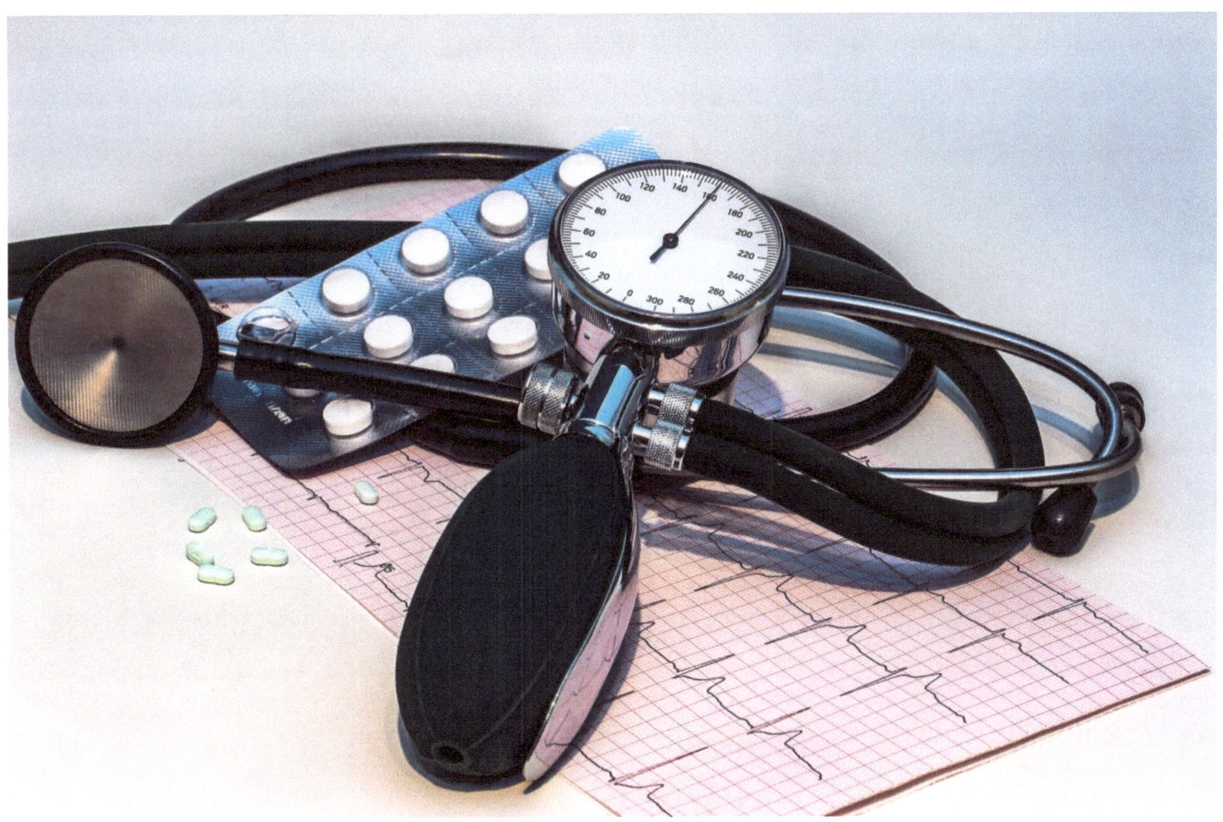

The greatest goal of this medication is to delay the onset of T1D, and it's worthwhile to discuss this treatment with your physician if you have the HLA-DQ8 trait.

Weight Loss and Diabetes

Before diving in, understand that remission of diabetes is not a cure. You should also understand that remission of diabetes is not possible with T1D. Only sustained lifestyle changes will maintain remission of T2D.

The best evidence of diabetic remission is through weight loss. Losing a mere five percent of your body weight can lead to remission. This was confirmed in a pilot study by McMaster University in Canada conducted to see if weight loss causes remission.

Eighty-three participants with T2D were placed on an 8- or 16-week intensive metabolic program combined with oral medication and lifestyle therapies to lose weight.

Forty percent of the participants managed to quit their medication at the end of the program. In addition, 28 individuals were still in remission after the three-month post-trial check-up.

Research performed at the University of Southern California successfully reversed T2D in mice with a fasting-mimicking diet, which includes minimal calories and fasting that promotes cellular regeneration to increase beta cells.

The most profound results came from the Diabetes Remission Clinical Trial (DiRECT), which found evidence of diabetes reversal in T2D. The UK study included 298 patients.

Participants were limited to no more than 850 calories a day over five months, and this included plenty of water, health shakes, and low-calorie soups.

Incredibly, 46% of the participants were in remission 12 months later, and 70% of these participants were still in remission 24 months later.

Participants who lost 22 pounds were successful after the first year. However, participants who lost 33 or more pounds were more successful in remission after the second year.

Remission was determined in patients who sustained long-term blood glucose levels of 48 millimoles per mole (mmol/mol).

Losing weight is undeniably the best way to reverse T2D.

Final Thoughts

Managing diabetes Type One or Two is becoming simpler with the research behind supplementary lifestyle and drug changes. Dropping a few pounds is never a bad idea.

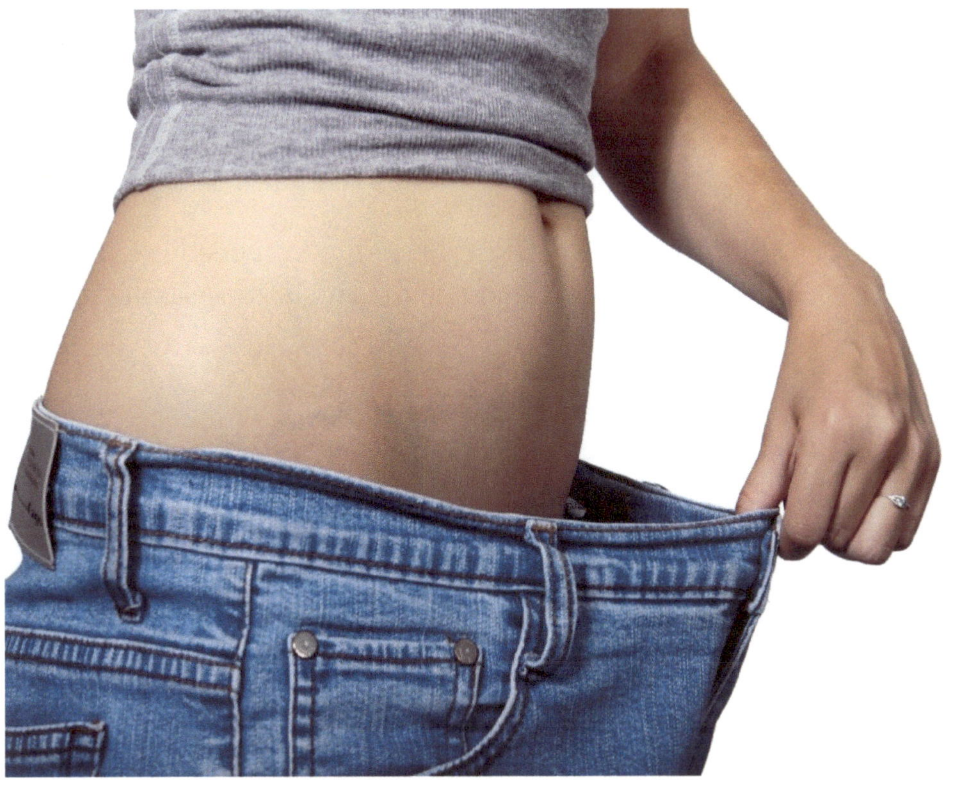

Diabetic Weight-Loss Tips and Tricks to Promote Remission

Type Two diabetes (T2D) is a chronic condition without a cure, and it happens when you become more and more resistant to insulin, which is supposed to regulate your blood glucose levels.

On a positive note, research into the main lifestyle change you need is exploding, proving that weight loss has the strongest evidence to promote remission. Saying it is one thing ... but losing weight must be carefully planned.

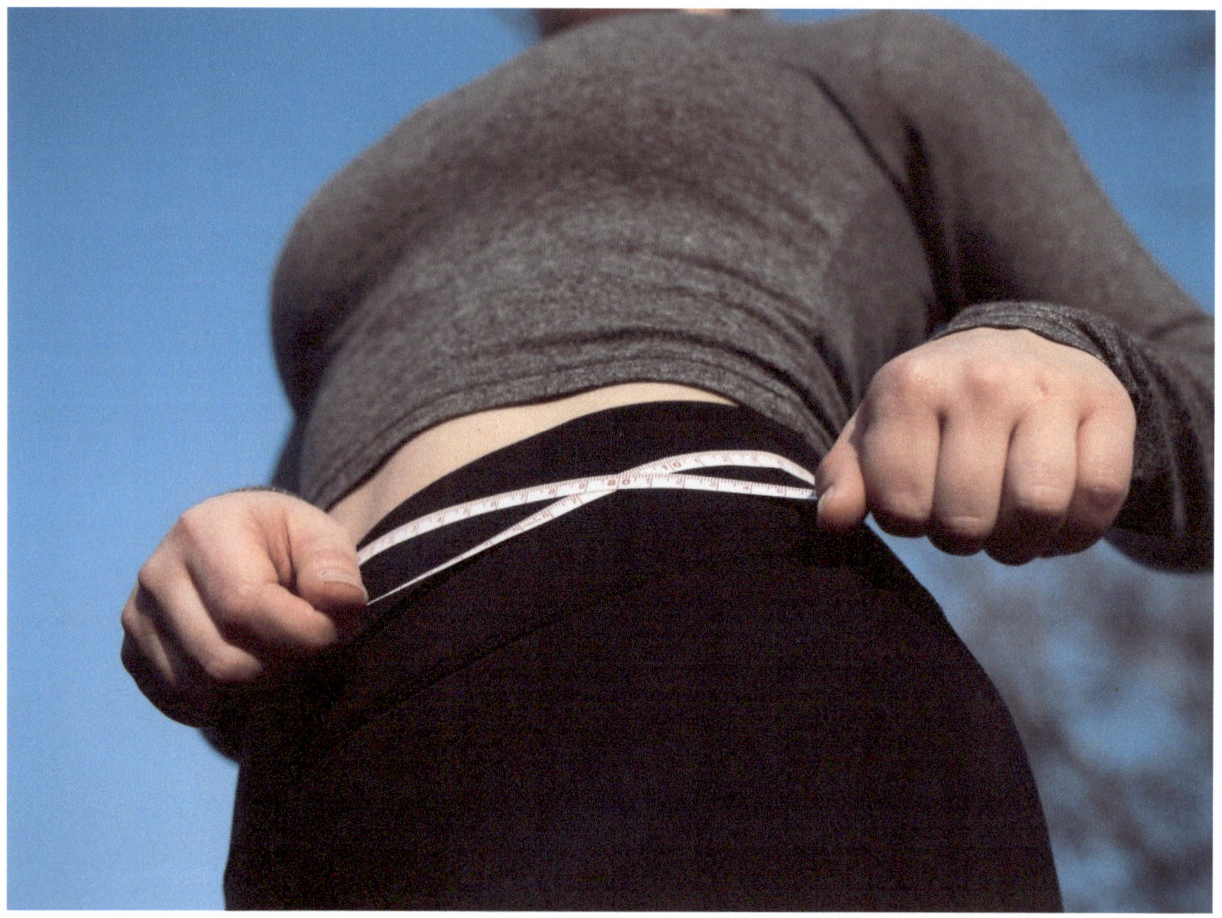

Weight-Loss Basics

Before jumping into a diet, understand where you're starting. Your body mass index (BMI), measurements, and current levels of fitness will help you design a better plan.

Calculating and Monitoring BMI

Your BMI places you in a category to indicate how overweight you are and how much weight you need to lose to reach the desired category. The categories for a BMI measurement are:

- 19 and under is underweight
- 19 to 24.9 is the sweet spot
- 25 to 29.9 is overweight
- 30 to 39.9 is obese
- 40 or more is morbidly obese

Medically, the target BMI for any person is the sweet spot. Make use of an online calculator to determine your BMI before you start losing weight, keep track of it for motivation as you progress, and use it to determine how much you should weigh.

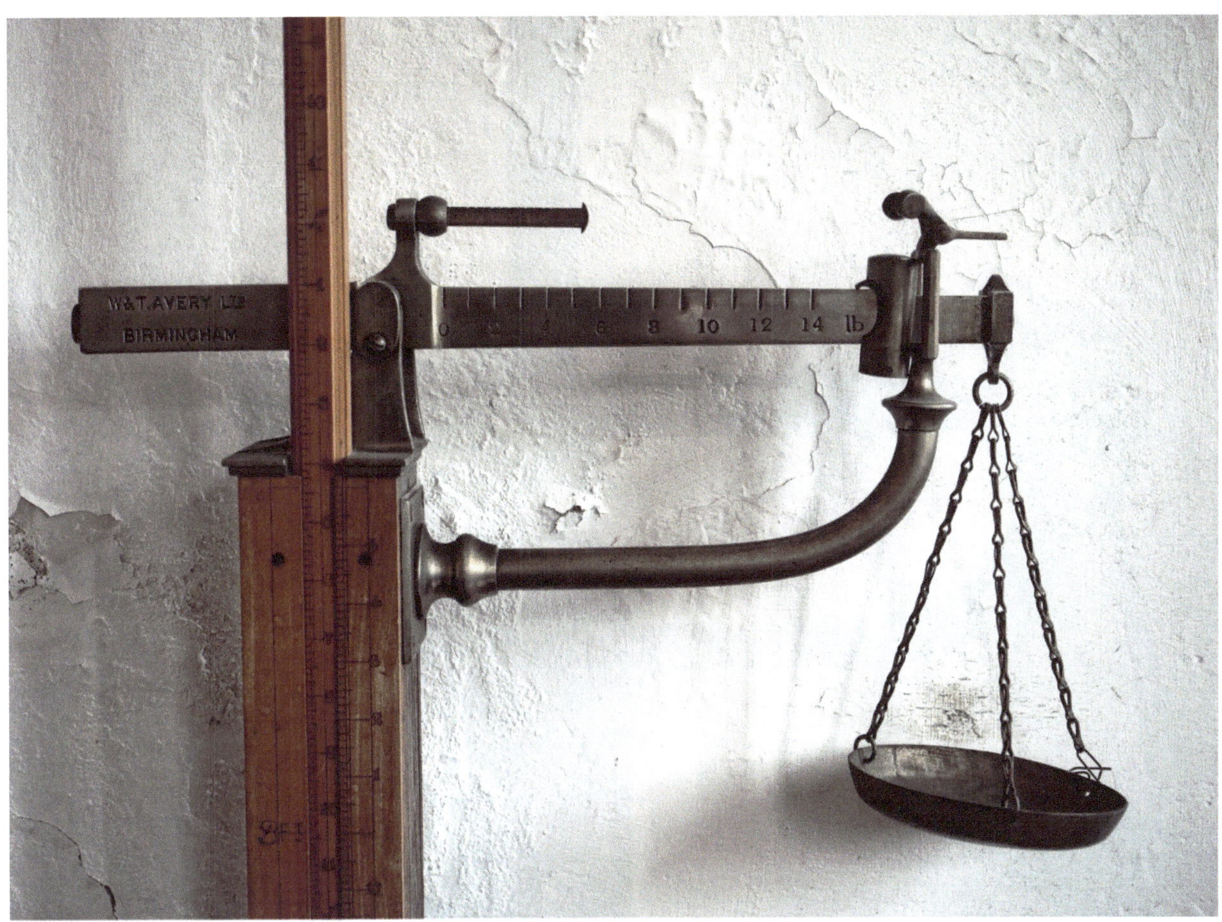

Measure Yourself

Sometimes, you won't see much movement on the scale, but measuring yourself gives you a more accurate result if you do it weekly. Take your initial measurements, write them in a diary, and keep measuring yourself weekly.

Determine Your Fitness

Your level of fitness determines how much exercise you can implement while you're on a low-calorie diet. Keep in mind that you need to balance the energy you spend with the energy you consume to achieve healthy weight loss.

The best way to determine whether you can implement strength or endurance training in your condition is to speak to your doctor. Your doctor may advise you to start with cardiovascular exercises before moving to the big fat burners.

The Low-Calorie Diet

Losing weight when you have diabetes can be achieved with the low-calorie option. The goal is to burn more calories than you consume daily, and that's why you need to know how fit you are.

Anything 1,200 calories or lower per day will require medical supervision. A low-calorie diet means you must avoid salt, refined carbohydrates, and trans fatty acids. These are the foods you aren't allowed to eat.

Instead, you'll be eating a lot of complex carbohydrates, lean proteins, and healthy fats, some of which are diabetic superfoods. Complex carbohydrates are balanced throughout the day with a low-calorie diet.

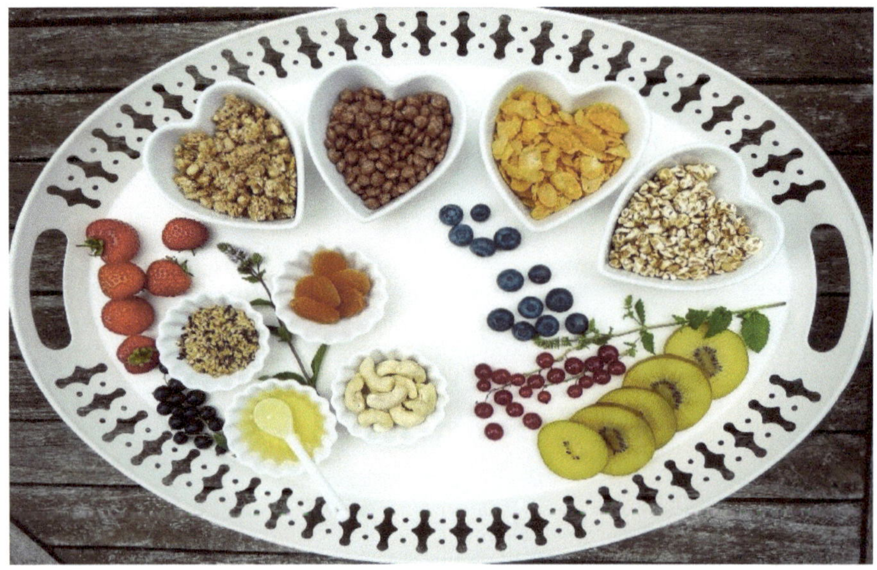

You'll have between 30 and 45 grams of carbohydrates with main meals and only 15 grams of carbs with snacks. The best way to ensure your correct carb and calorie intake is to make a seven-day meal plan every week.

Buy a kitchen scale to stick to your measured portions daily and use an online calorie calculator to find out the number of calories in each food Type and portion size.

You can also use another online calculator to determine how many calories you should be eating daily. Always remember to discuss your calorie intake with a medical professional first.

The best ingredients on a low-calorie diet include broccoli, salmon, raw nuts, beans, cinnamon, organic oatmeal, dairy, quinoa, olive oil, and spinach. Be sure to add a few low-calorie ingredients to special soups and shakes, and drink plenty of water.

Burn Fat with Exercise

The power of movement has many benefits for diabetics, but exercise is also a guaranteed method of losing weight. You'll have to kick it up a notch if you want to burn calories and fat.

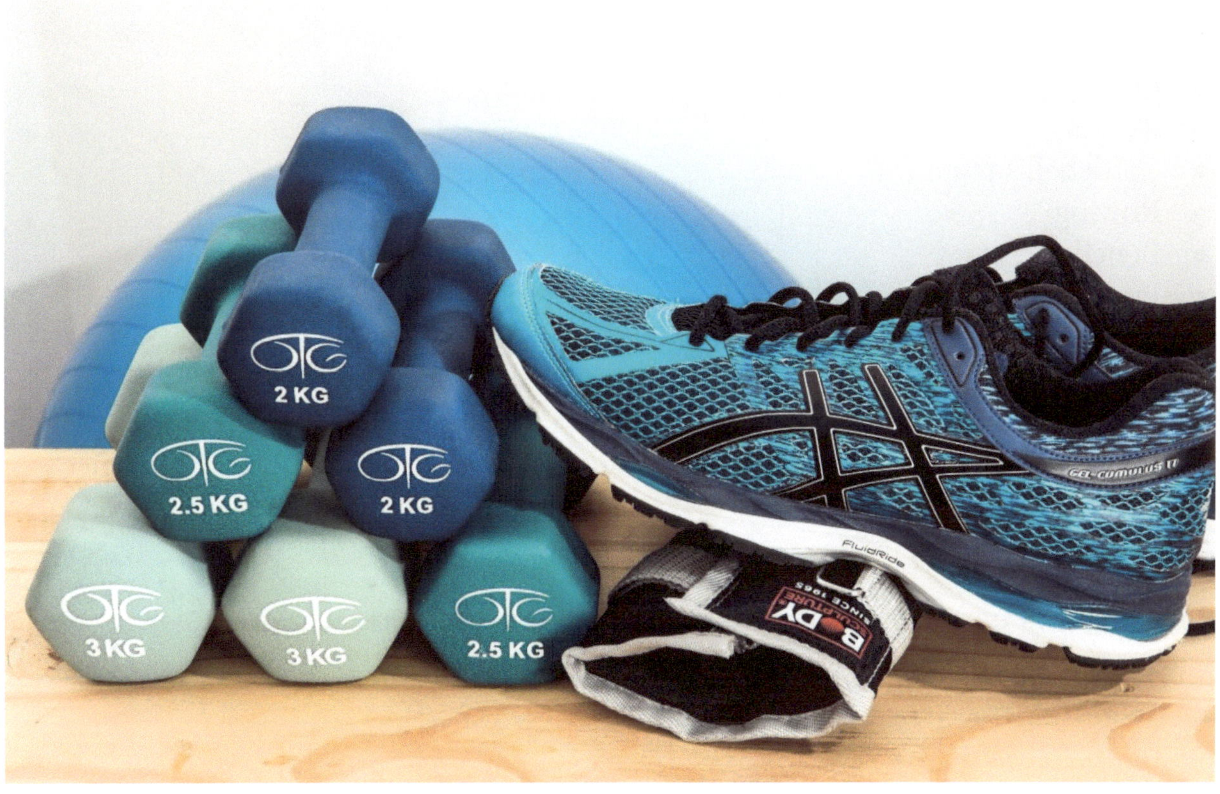

To lose weight, you need to exercise moderately for 30 minutes a day, five times per week. You can also divide this time throughout the day, such as exercising for three 10-minute sessions daily.

Cardio Options

Cardiovascular workouts can help you lose weight if they're more than a slow walk in the park. They include:

- Cycling
- Running
- Swimming
- Brisk walking
- Jogging
- Aerobics
- Spinning
- Elliptical Training
- Kickboxing

Strength Training

A study by Wake Forest University confirmed that weight training is better than cardio workouts if you intend to lose weight. This might include:

- Lifting weights
- Push-ups
- Squats
- Kettlebell squats
- Rowing
- Bench presses
- Pull-ups
- Dumbbells
- Stair climbing
- Sprawls Resistance band training

Whatever exercise routine you choose, make sure you discuss it with your doctor first.

A Weight-Loss Secret

Losing weight is hard, so consider doing it with a friend. Social factors play a role in diabetes management, so enlist a weight-loss buddy to guarantee success.

Final Thoughts

Eating fewer calories and becoming active indeed gives you a chance of pushing your T2D into remission where it belongs. Lowering your BMI brings immense benefits, which you'll notice in more than your blood glucose levels.

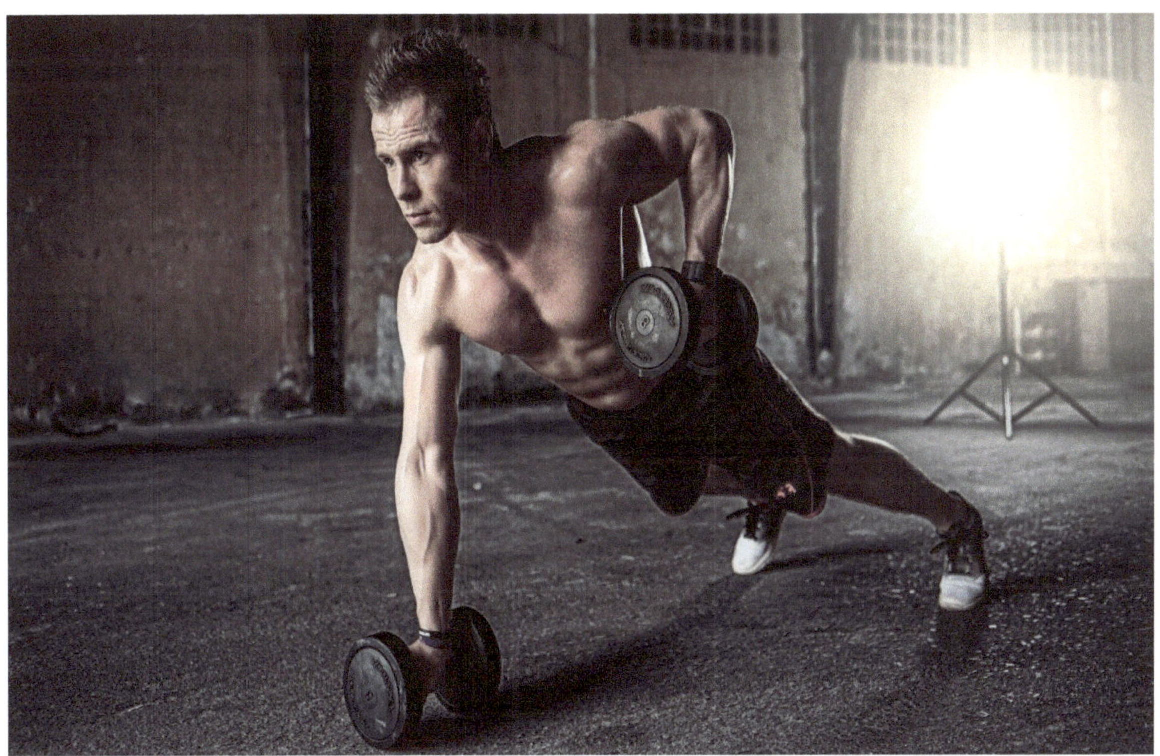

Basic Reminders for Caring for Type Two Diabetes at Home

Maybe you or a loved one was just diagnosed with Type Two diabetes (T2D). Or perhaps you've been struggling with it for years. Either way, it's hard to be diagnosed with a chronic condition.

It changes your psychological landscape and keeping the condition under control seems impossible. Truthfully, insulin resistance is reversible and manageable through simple changes that can also prevent complications.

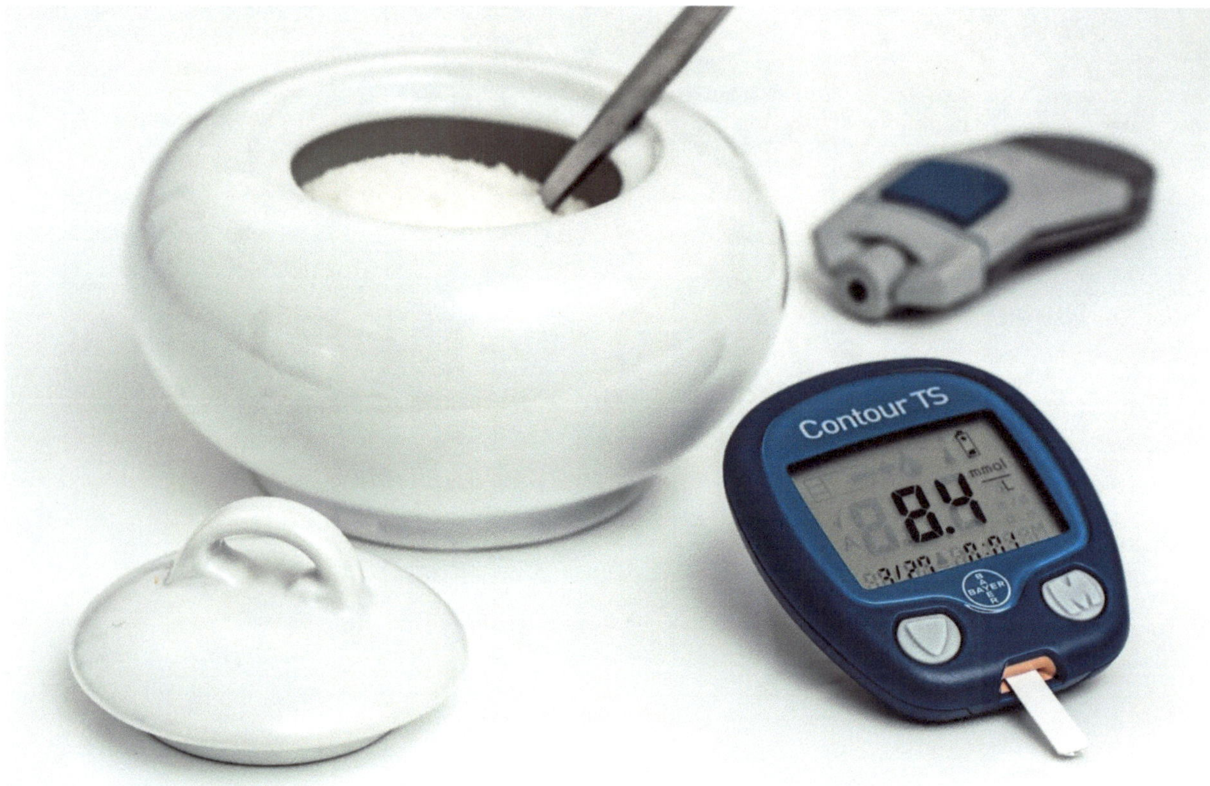

Quick Basics

T2D is a lifelong condition where cell receptors become resistant to insulin even though the pancreas continues to produce it. Pancreatic beta cells release insulin to allow other cells in your body to collect, convert, and store energy.

The cells in the liver and muscles have a layer of mitochondria that exposes itself through insulin absorption, and it turns carbohydrates into glucose.

With too many carbs, the cells become overworked, but the pancreas continues to produce insulin. Eventually, the mitochondria stop functioning as they should.

Tracking Your Blood Glucose Levels

Insulin resistance can worsen if it's unmonitored. Make sure you have a blood glucose meter with lancets and test strips to keep an eye on your glucose levels when you wake up, before meals, an hour after meals, and at bedtime.

A normal fasting blood glucose reading is between 71 and 140 milligrams per deciliter (mg/dL). Anything lower is *hypo*glycemia, and anything higher is *hyper*glycemia, both of which are dangerous.

What Causes Fluctuations?

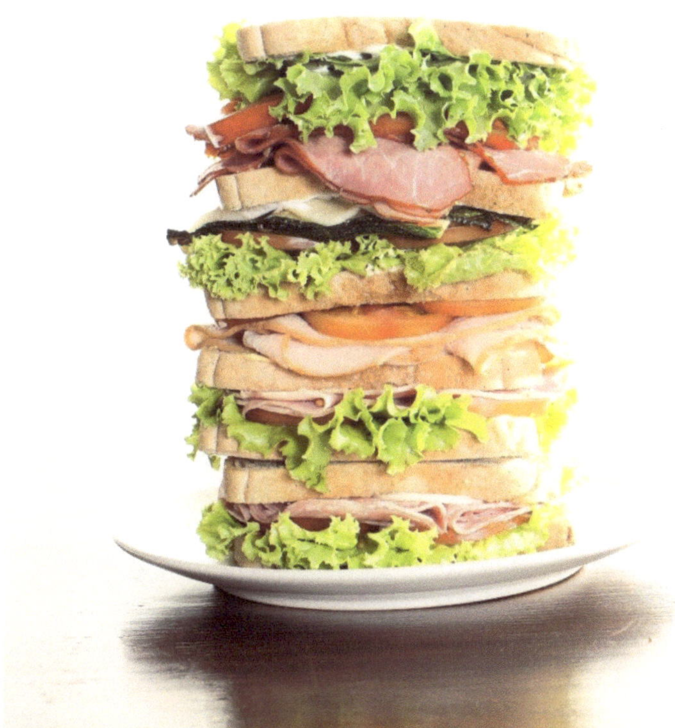

A few things can cause your blood glucose to spike, such as:

- Eating too many carbohydrates, especially the simple ones
- Eating very large meals
- Skipping your medication
- Not exercising
- Stress, pain, and other illnesses

- Sunburn
- Skipping breakfast
- A lack of sleep
- The dawn phenomenon (your blood glucose levels spike around 3:00 AM)
- Dehydration
- Menstrual cycles
- Steroids and antipsychotic medication side effects

Certain things also cause hypoglycemia, such as:

- Not eating enough or missing meals

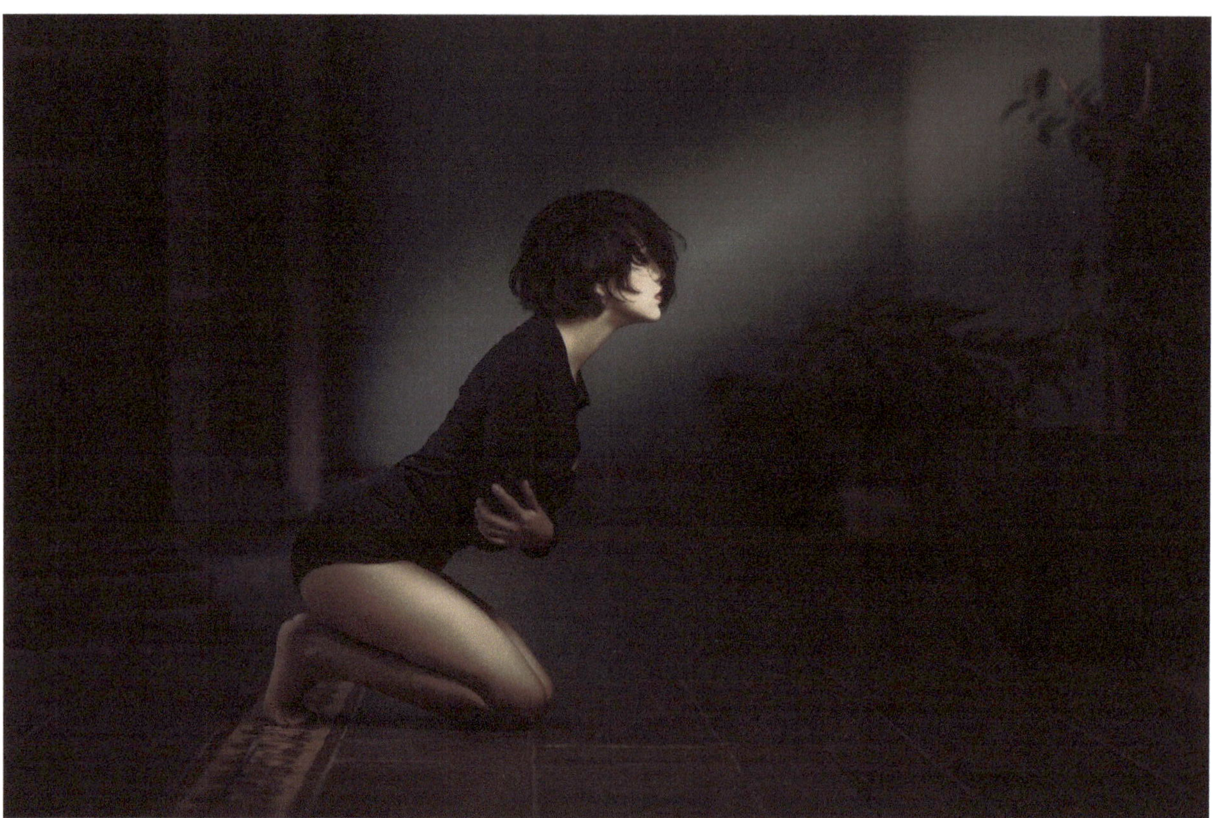

- Reducing your carbohydrate intake too much
- Alcohol
- Taking too high of a dose of your diabetic medication
- Too much physical activity (exercise routines should always be discussed with your doctor)
- Side effects from other medications
- Hormone deficiencies

Quick Balancing Acts

Blood glucose that's ***too high*** or low can cause serious complications, so you want to restore balance.

Some ways to bring blood glucose down fast are:

- Drink two glasses of water
- Exercise
- Drink green tea
- Drink black coffee
- Seek medical attention if levels remain high

What to do if your blood glucose is ***too low***:

1. Eat or drink something with fast-acting sugar, albeit a small amount

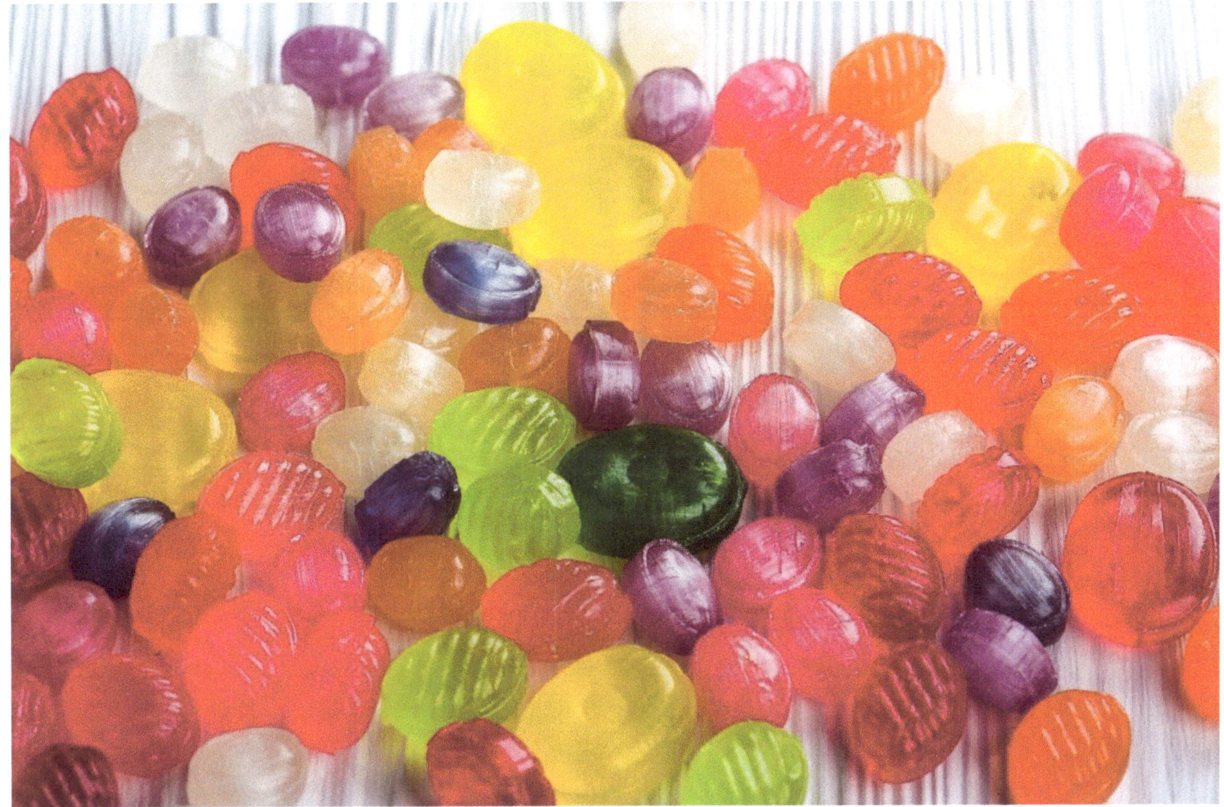

2. Wait 10 minutes
3. Test your glucose again
4. Seek medical attention if your levels remain low

Two Main Homecare Reminders

Two changes in your daily life can help you maintain better control and even reverse the condition. Remission isn't a cure; it's the temporary reversal of a condition, and it's up to you to keep it that way.

Maintaining Weight Loss

Weight loss is the best management strategy for T2D. Evidence suggests that it can cause remission in diabetic patients, but remission is temporary and controlled by your daily lifestyle, which means that you need to maintain the weight loss.

A longitudinal study of 33,184 participants over 23 years was published in the *BMC Public Health Journal*. The subjects were all at high risk of developing T2D, and the majority of their body mass indices (BMIs) were nearly normal at 25.

Over the years, those who didn't maintain their BMI had an increase in their risk for diabetes. The risk increased by between 1.04 and 1.06% every time the participants gained one percent of their body weight.

Weight maintenance is associated with better management. The accumulation of fat around the liver and pancreas leads to your beta cells not working properly, which could cause insulin resistance or the eventual need for insulin.

A review by Newcastle University examined the likelihood of staying in remission with fast weight loss and maintenance. According to the review, many diabetics lose weight, but they quickly regain it over the first year.

This yo-yo effect doesn't decrease the long-term risks of the condition returning. According to the Diabetes Remission Clinical Trial (DiRECT), maintenance should follow a loss of 33 pounds.

Using a low-calorie diet with physical activity helps you melt the fat around your liver and pancreas, but maintaining it requires you to stick to a healthier lifestyle and avoid returning to old habits.

Participants of numerous studies in the review were more successful in long-term remission when they maintained their weight loss. Some of them maintained remission for 5 and 10 years.

Don't simply aim to lose weight; use diabetic-friendly lifestyle changes to keep your risk at bay.

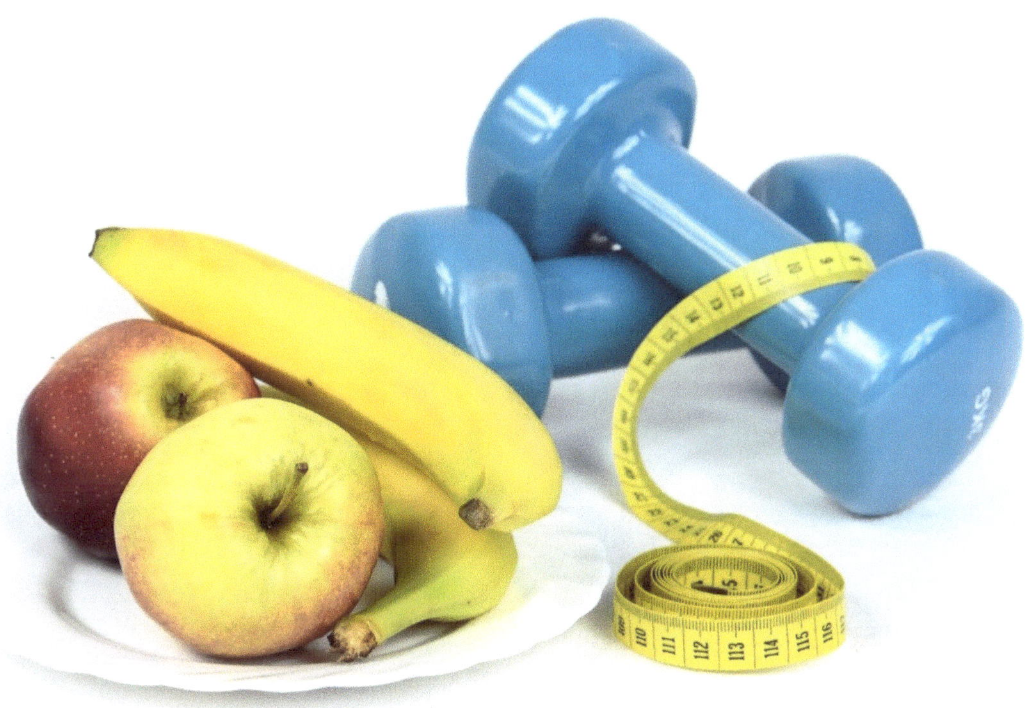

Psychological Battle

Finding out that you have a lifelong condition takes its toll on your psychological well-being. Stress is natural when you don't know how to manage your condition or reverse it. Unfortunately, the stress hormones cortisol and adrenaline aggravate T2D.

They cause uncontrollable fluctuations in blood glucose, impair glucose and insulin tolerance, and activate fat cells. Stress even pushes your blood pressure up, causing your risk for heart disease to increase.

The only way to avoid this is by dealing with your stress daily. Some useful methods to reduce stress include:

- Journaling
- Meditation
- Mindfulness
- Socializing
- Exercise
- Laughing more
- Learning more about diabetes
- Eating healthier
- Sleeping better
- Talking to a professional
- Removing stress triggers
- Practicing progressive muscle relaxation (PMR)

- Using breathing exercises
- Organizing your days

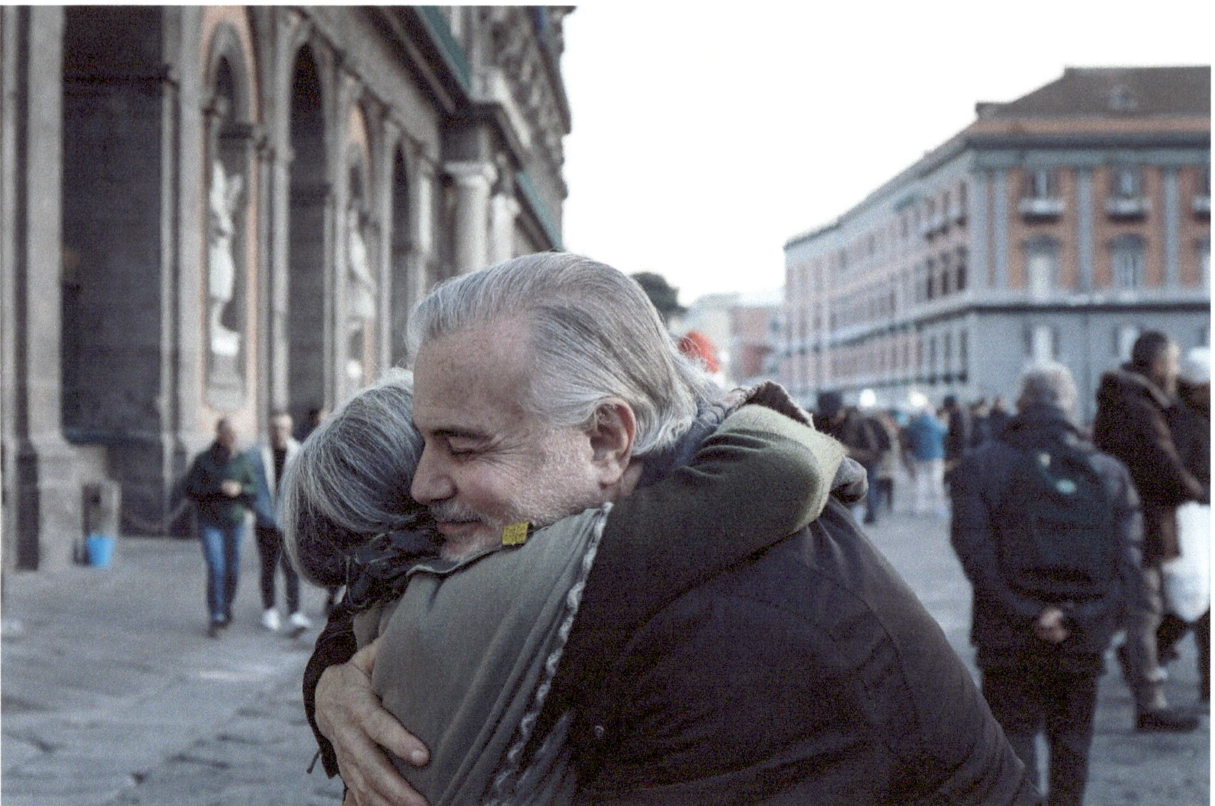

- Taking a nature walk
- Hugging someone
- Getting a new hobby
- Setting SMART goals
- Adopting optimism
- Practicing positive self-talk
- Expressing gratitude
- Joining a yoga class

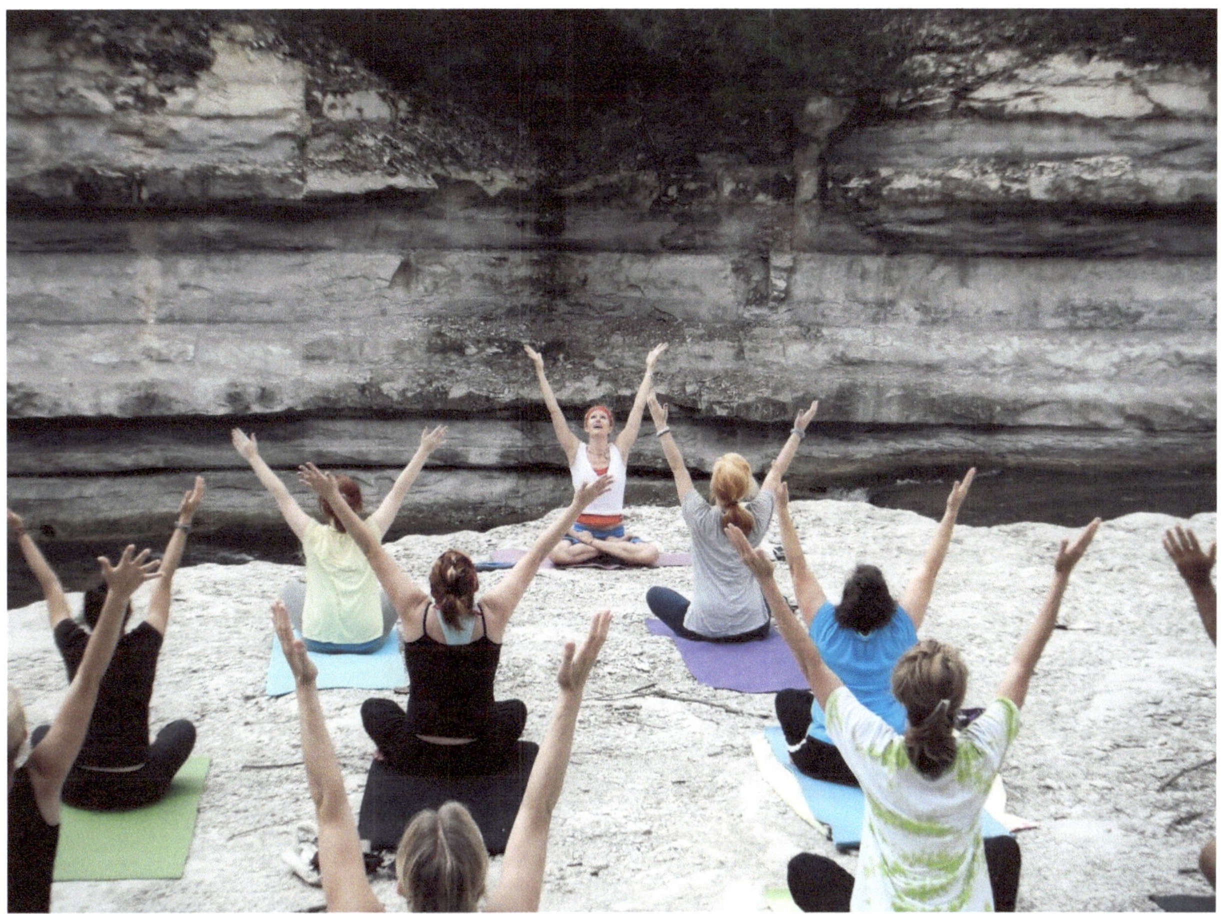

Living under stress only makes the battle harder. Adopt a few new habits to counteract the consequences of uncontrolled T2D.

Final Thoughts

Managing your T2D at home is simple with the right knowledge, weight loss to keep your condition under control, and stress-reducing techniques to make your days a little easier.

Controlling Type One Diabetes at Home Requires Knowledge

Finding out that you or your child has Type One diabetes (T1D) is something no one wants to hear. The thought of being dependent on insulin by injection or pump can be overwhelming, even though it's your best line of defense.

The biotech industry is making progress on the battlefield against T1D and constantly looking for a cure, and they're making diabetes management less overwhelming in the meantime.

Some advancements even offer a glimpse of hope that a cure is close at hand. In the meantime, the best way you can prevent complications is to learn more about insulin.

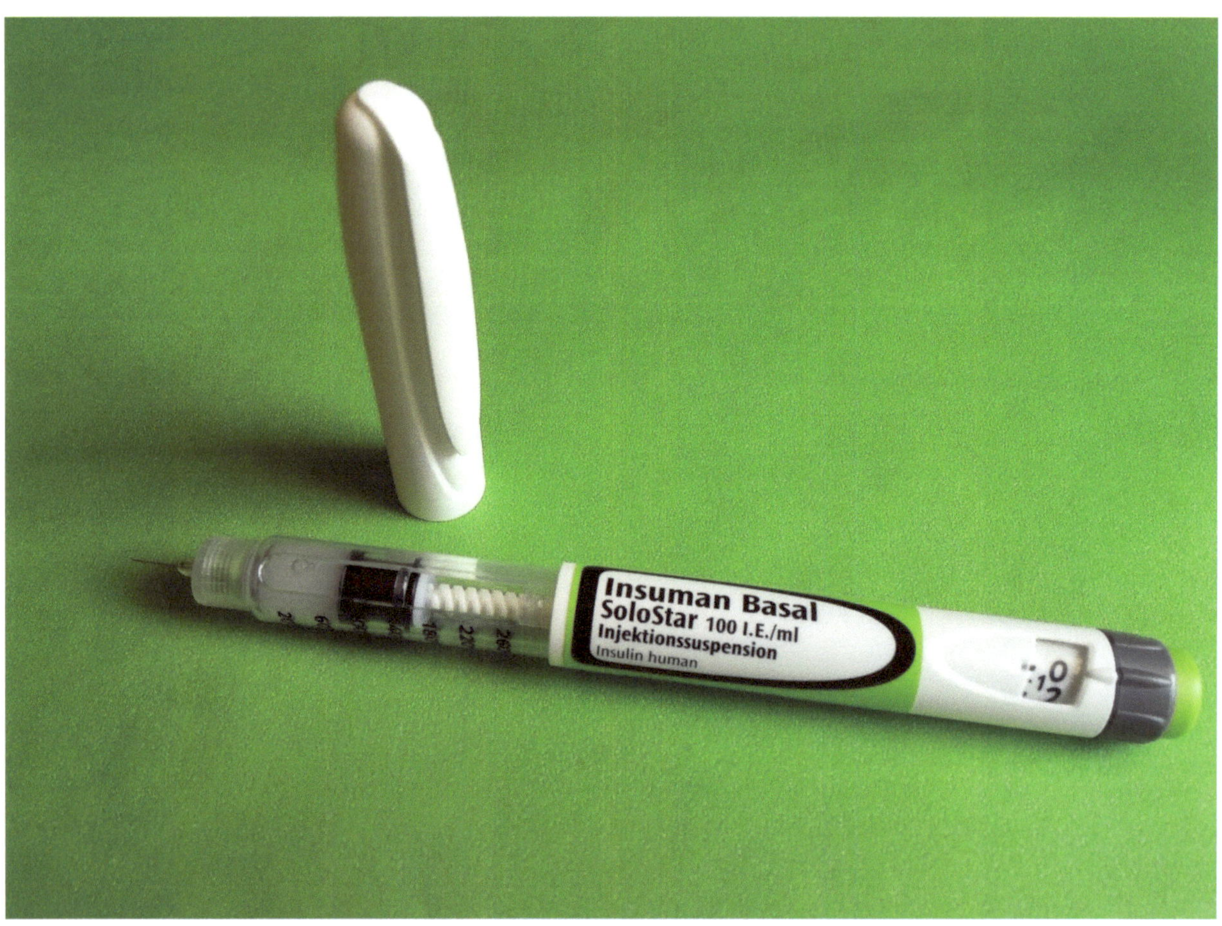

A T1D Breakdown

Children are the most affected by T1D because its onset is different from Type Two. Individuals don't have control of their risk for T1D. An autoimmune malfunction is the cause as the body's immune system turns insulin-producing cells into the enemy.

The immune system goes to battle against the pancreatic beta cells, depleting them completely in some cases. Without beta cells, the body can't produce insulin to regulate blood glucose anymore, which leads to uncontrolled glucose levels.

The person with Type One diabetes becomes dependent on external insulin to manage their condition.

Insulin Evolution

Your child might've been diagnosed recently, and your fear as a parent is justified, especially if you don't know much about insulin management. Fortunately, the evolution of insulin has made it a lot safer and more efficient.

Paul Langerhans was the founder of a cluster of cells within the pancreas in 1869. These are the cells responsible for insulin production, and the clusters were later named the Islets of Langerhans.

In 1901, American Physician Eugene Opie was the first man to discover that the destruction of these cells caused diabetes because the body can no longer produce its own insulin.

In 1921, Frederick Banting and Charles Best from Toronto, Canada, started experimenting successfully by injecting liquidized pancreas into dogs with T1D, and by 1922, they helped a boy with T1D live 13 years.

Eli Lilly was the first manufacturer to produce fast-acting insulin in 1922, and intermediate insulin was found by Novo Nordisk in 1950. The first human synthesized insulin became available through biotechnology in 1978.

This was a huge step forward in insulin safety because allergic reactions were less common with the synthesis from human cells. Previously, cells taken from an animal pancreas were often rejected by the human immune system.

But now, insulin was safer for children and young adults globally. The evolution sprung forward from this point.

Injections were another unpleasant part of insulin therapy, and the insulin pen was released by Novo Nordisk in 1985. It provided better accuracy, easier use, and less injection pain.

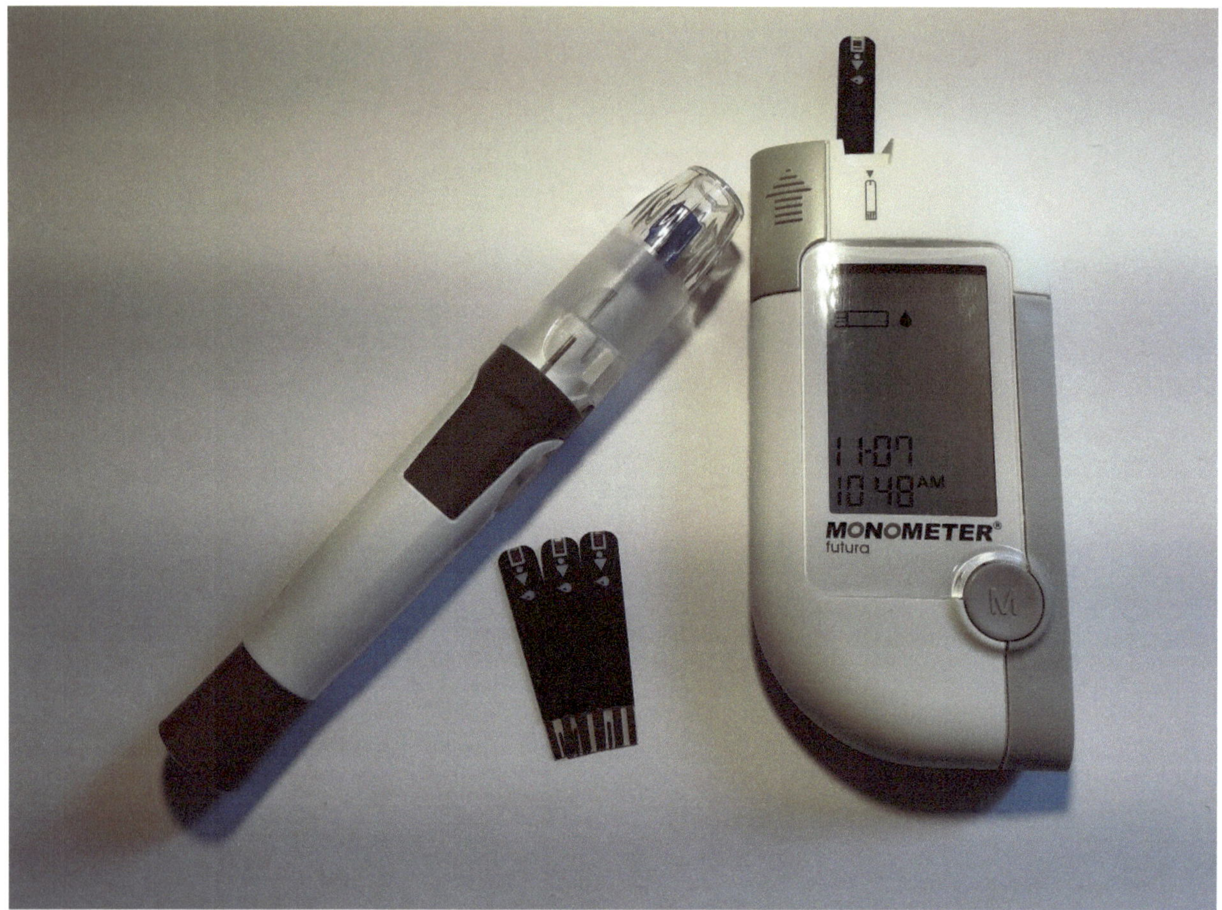

Medtronic released the first insulin pump in 1992, called the MiniMed 506. It was an incredible leap forward in T1D treatment. The MiniMed 506 could deliver insulin for daily requirements, and by using a meal bolus memory, it delivered precise doses of insulin two hours after eating.

Eli Lilly introduced genetically-modified insulin in 1996, called Humalog. The amino acids in Humalog have been altered to improve absorption, distribution, metabolism, and excretion, making it more effective than previous insulins.

The 21st century saw a flood of new advancements, including an artificial pancreas with glucose monitors.

Whether you're using a pump or injectable human insulin, the synthesized hormone has become much safer if you follow guidelines from your doctor.

The Different Types of Insulin

There are four main types of insulin, namely:

- Rapid-acting insulin, which works in 15 minutes and lasts three to four hours. This is the one you often use before meals.
- Short-acting insulin, which works in 30 to 60 minutes and lasts for five to eight hours. It's also often used before meals.
- Intermediate-acting insulin, which works in one to two hours and lasts for 14 to 16 hours.
- Long-acting insulin, which works after two hours and lasts 24 hours or more.

Best Injection Sites

Your healthcare provider will show you how to inject insulin subcutaneously. The best sites for injectable insulin are:

- Abdomen
- Upper arms
- Upper thighs
- Buttocks

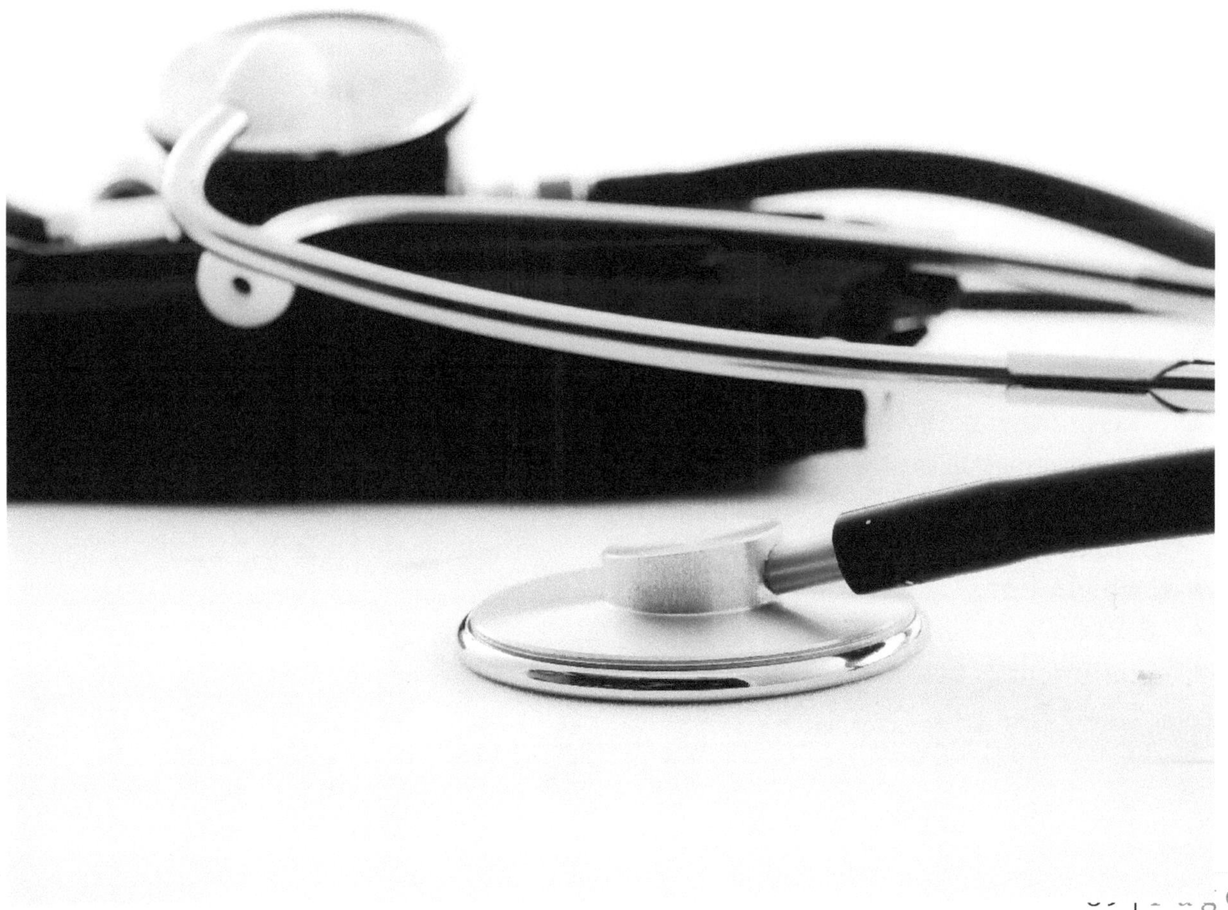

Insulin Reaction

Sometimes, you might have a reaction to insulin, which most often manifests in hypoglycemia, an extremely low blood glucose level. Symptoms might include:

- Fatigue
- Sweating
- Confusion
- Loss of consciousness
- Seizures
- Inability to speak
- Pale skin
- Muscle twitches

How to Stop the Reaction

Anyone using insulin should carry with them 15 grams of fast-acting carbohydrates at all times. This might be half a cup of fruit juice, two tablespoons of raisins, one tablespoon of honey, or five lifesaver candies.

Ironically, lifesaver candies are the easiest fast-acting carbohydrate to carry, and they can save you or your child's life. Additionally, ensure that everyone knows of your child's condition and how to help them if you're not around.

Beware of the Insulin Saboteurs

Insulin use is simple with your doctor's instructions, but some habits could sabotage your management. They include:

- Forgetting to measure your glucose levels
- Missing a dose
- Skipping meals
- Making unhealthy food choices
- Allowing stress into your life
- Not exercising
- Smoking
- Dehydration
- Being overweight
- Continuously injecting insulin in the same spot

Avoid these problems to keep your insulin therapy at optimum effect.

Final Thoughts

Managing your T1D or that of your child becomes less stressful when you learn a few details about your treatment. Insulin is much safer than it used to be, which can reduce stress while getting used to a new treatment method. Make sure to discuss any problems or questions with your doctor.

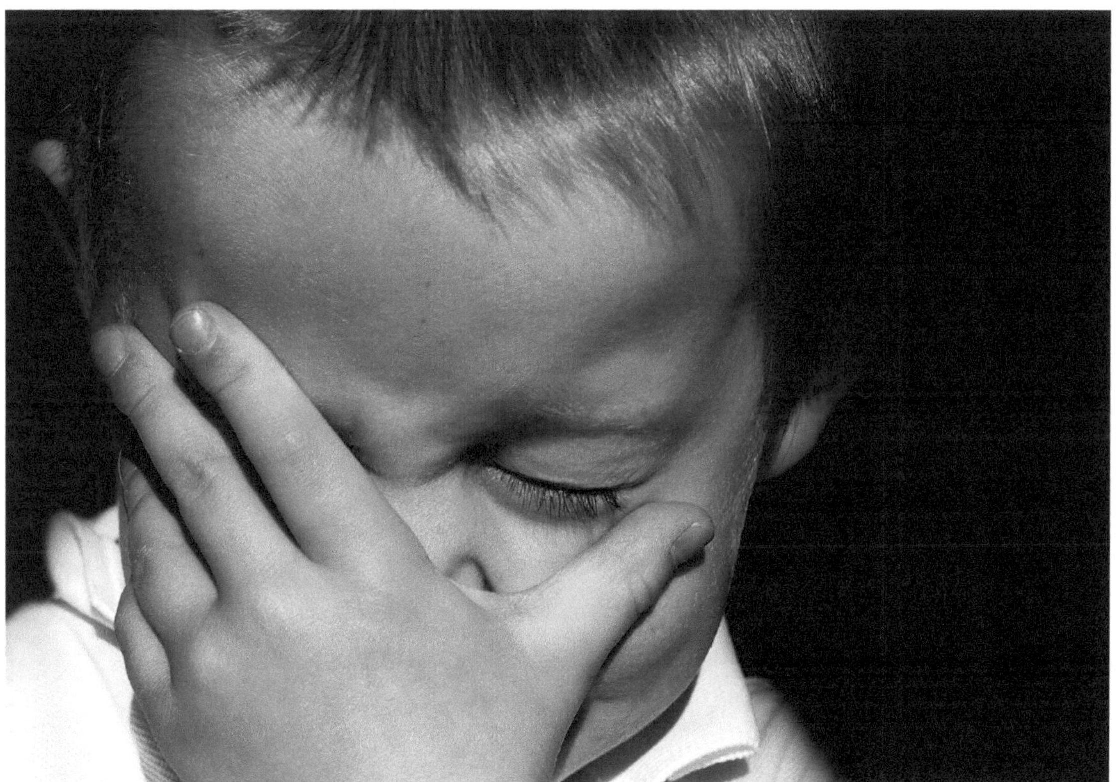

A Few Diabetes Concerns Came to Light Through Research

Humans are responsible for the way they respond to life, but it's quite difficult to control the environment's impact on our health and our medical conditions such as diabetes.

It's well known that the wrong foods can overwork our immune systems, and some can even destroy the natural helpers found in the stomach.

However, there are two significant threats in the world, and learning about them changes the way you manage Type One (T1D) or Type Two diabetes (T2D).

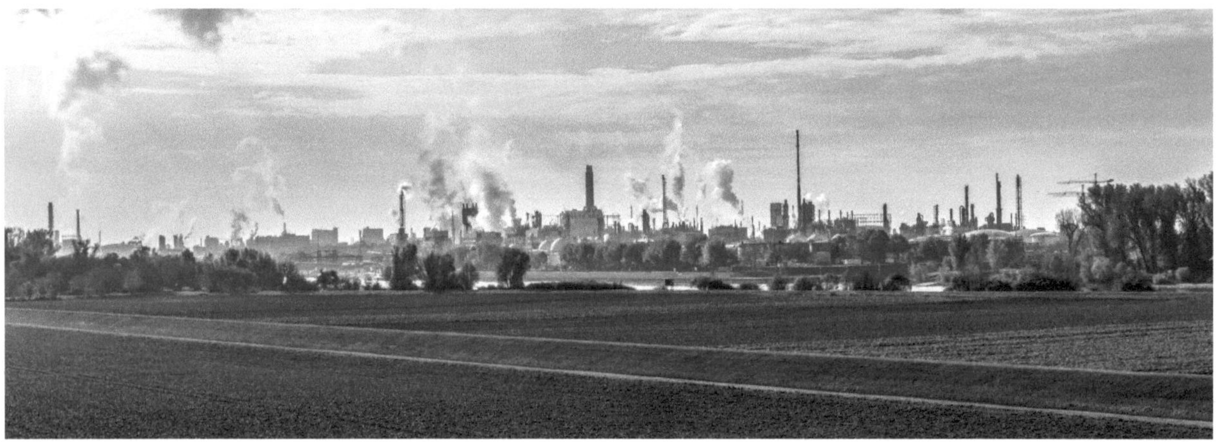

Environmental Threats

Type One diabetes' causational factors are debatable, but it's an autoimmune disorder where the immune system distinguishes beta cells in the pancreas as threats and destroys them. These beta cells are required for insulin production.

In developing treatment or even a cure for an autoimmune disorder, researchers try to answer the question of why it occurs. In several cases, T1D develops in children who had diseases such as mumps, measles, and other viral infections.

The incidence of T1D has increased over the last few decades, and the question has arisen as to what effect the industrialization of our environment may have had.

Associate Professor Mihaela Stefan-Lifshitz from the Albert Einstein College of Medicine found that common chemical exposure and genetic factors are collectively correlating with increases in numbers.

Exposure to environmental chemicals can damage the beta cells in your pancreas, and it is suspected that this damage could influence the development of T1D in some people.

Environmental chemicals include mercury, lead, asbestos, formaldehyde, air pollutants, pesticides like glyphosate, polychlorinated biphenyls (BPAs), and poly-fluoroalkyl substances (PFAs).

Formaldehyde

This chemical is found in many construction and household products, such as adhesives, plywood, permanent-press fabrics, and insulation materials. It's a colorless and pungent gas used in building materials.

A study published by the Aston University in Birmingham showed that formaldehyde is correlated with increased risk for T2D, dementia, and depression.

Mercury

Mercury is another chemical commonly used in fluorescent lamps, medicine, and thermometers, and it can cause beta cell abnormalities in the pancreas, which can lead to an increased risk of diabetes.

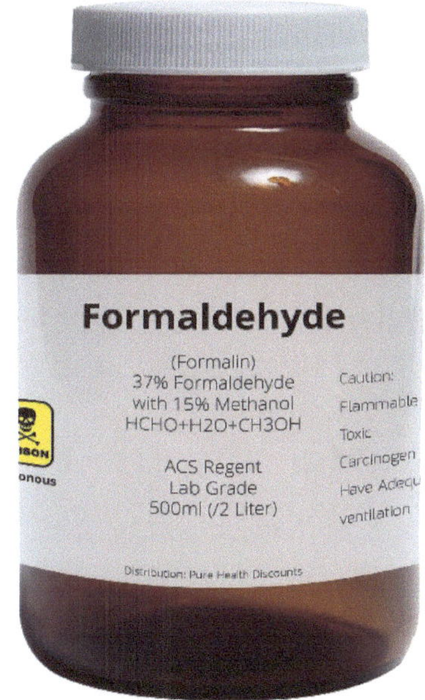

This chemical is found in non-organic farm products. It's an herbicide used to reduce damage from pests and speed up the harvesting process. A study of nearly 2,000 Thai farmers concluded that exposure to glyphosate was associated with diabetes occurrence.

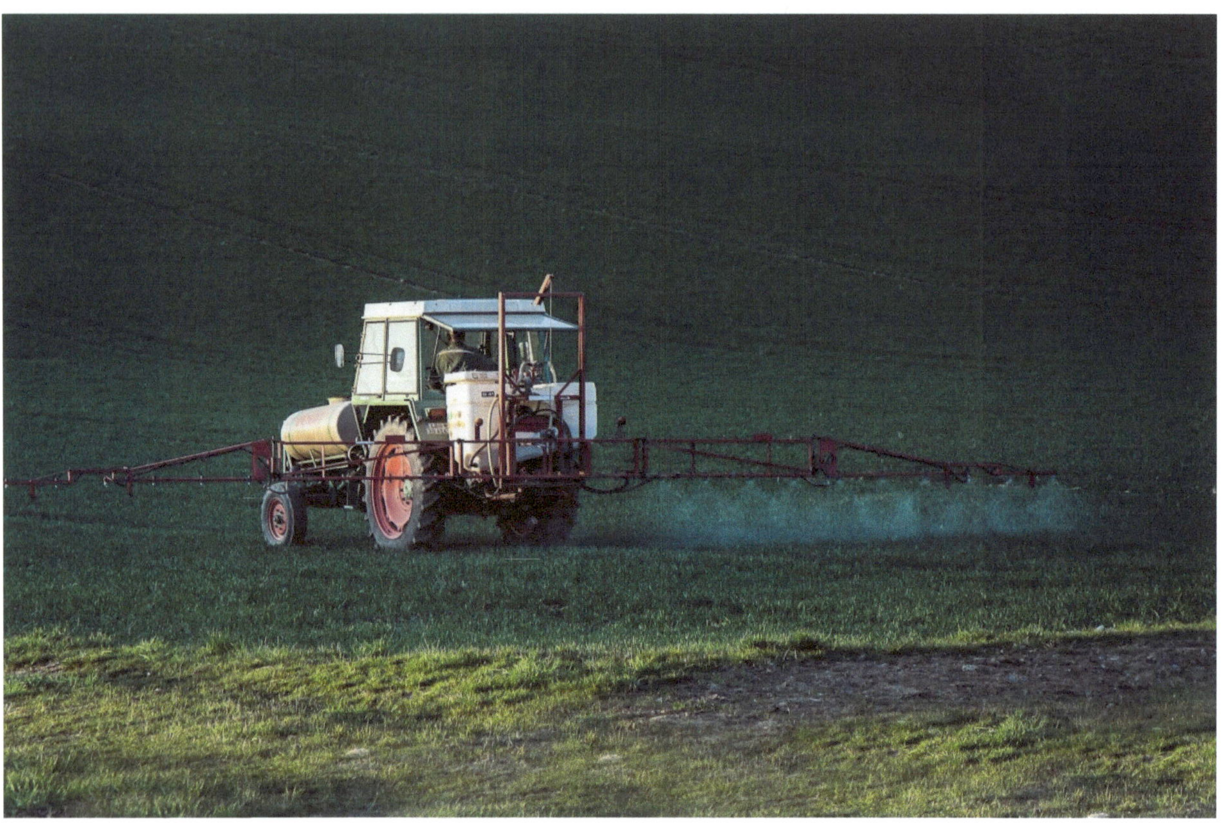

Stress

Stress is the second factor increasing your risk for diabetes. Also, it can be a consequence of diabetes. If you think about it, stress can be categorized as another environmental factor.

Linkoping University in Sweden published a study that correlated childhood stress with an increased risk of developing T1D because of the impact stress has on hormones and the immune system.

A review published by the European Depression in Diabetes (EDID) Research Consortium confirms that elevated levels of daily stress also correlate with the development of T2D.

__Understanding the Stress Response__

Stress is a physical response occurring when you feel threatened. The pituitary glands in the brain instruct the release of cortisol and epinephrine from the adrenal glands near your kidneys.

The fight-or-flight response is psychologically triggered, and this is the stress response understood by most people. What you might not know is that the pancreas, liver, and digestive systems also respond.

Cells have two receptors, one to release insulin and another to store glucose. Stored glucose is released in the form of glucagon during acute stress responses so that the body has the energy to combat a threat. This explains why blood glucose levels and blood pressure rise quickly under stress.

Glucagon should be reserved for times of starvation, which is another internal threat to the body, but it's also released when you need to be alert and ready to face a threat. This is a response that is supposed to be protective for the body, but sometimes this "response" can happen too often.

When occasional stress becomes chronic stress, the glucagon release occurs much more often. This frequent release of the glucagon depletes your resources, and the cells become overworked.

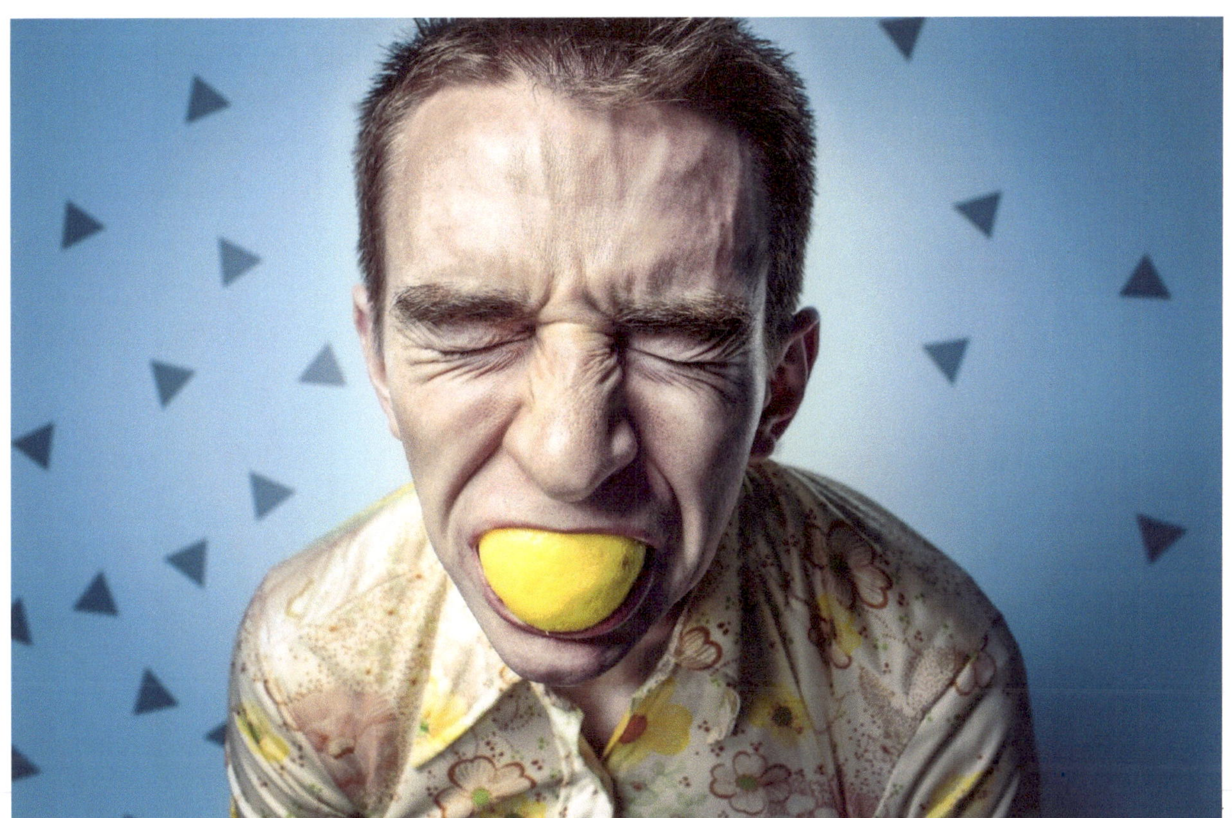

Either the cell receptors become resistant to insulin as in T2D, or the pancreatic beta cells that produce insulin overwork themselves until they stop working as in T1D.

Stress is a massive factor in the risk of developing diabetes.

Final Thoughts

Being aware of the dangers in the environment, including stress, helps you navigate a healthier life. Limiting your exposure to environmental toxins is the best decision.

Chronic Kidney Disease and Treatment

If the information in this book benefited you by helping better control your diabetes, then you may be interested in one of my other books – ***Chronic Kidney Disease Management and Treatment*** - *https://www.amazon.com/dp/B0915M63FC*.

It too was written by the same ER Physician with 25 years of experience and training. Kidney Disease, diabetes and high blood pressure all seem to go hand in hand and if you have one, you may have one (or both) of the other two. If you have chronic kidney disease, my other book will help you manage and control it too.

Like this book, it too is teaming with up-to-date information on how to better manage and treat chronic kidney disease – a common disease associated with diabetes.

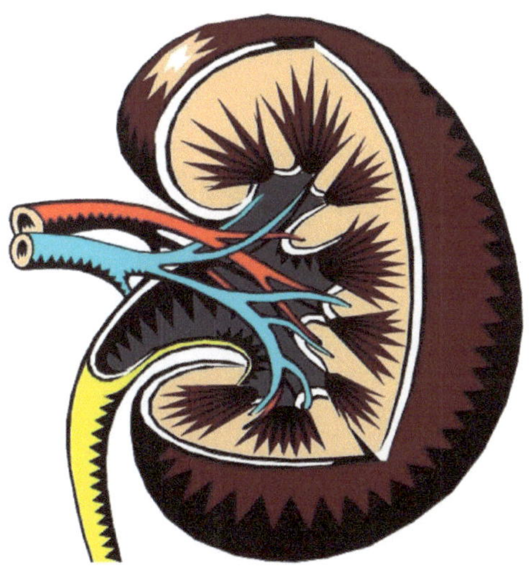

https://www.amazon.com/dp/B0915M63FC

About the Author

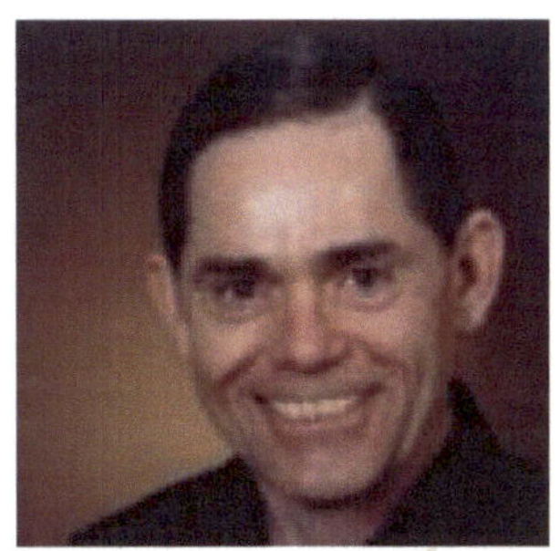

I am a published writer with numerous books on Amazon for Kindle and other publishing platforms … both in electronic and Print On Demand (POD) formats.

While most of my self-published books are on health and fitness in general, my topics of interest currently are more toward 1) aging baby boomers and the older population and 2) low content books, like word activity books, journals, planners and calendars.

Besides my own writing, I also ghost-write ebooks, books, reports, articles, autoresponder series, blogs and Kindle conversions for my client base on a variety of topics. I'm currently using Microsoft's Office Suite including Word, PowerPoint and Publisher, along with Affinity Publisher and Designrr for writing and publishing.

Go to my website at http://ronknesswriting.com for more information or to request a quote: https://ronknesswriting.com/ghostwriting-quote-request-form.

For a complete list of my books published on Amazon, go to https://www.amazon.com/Ron-Kness/e/B0072M6PYO.

Today my wife and I are retired from our careers and live in Queen Creek, AZ. I now write as a retirement business where you'll find me happily sitting in my office typing away on my computer as I work on my next book or ghostwriting project for a client . . . that is if we are not traveling somewhere in our RV - our renewed mode of travel.

Take care and be safe!

Ron